MOTIVATIONAL INTERVIEWING WITH FAMILIES

Applications of Motivational Interviewing
Stephen Rollnick, William R. Miller,
and Theresa B. Moyers, Series Editors

Since the publication of Miller and Rollnick's classic *Motivational Interviewing*, now in its fourth edition, MI has been widely adopted as a tool for facilitating change. This highly practical series includes general MI resources as well as books on specific clinical contexts, problems, and populations. Each volume presents powerful MI strategies that are grounded in research and illustrated with concrete, "how-to-do-it" examples.

RECENT VOLUMES

Motivational Interviewing in Health Care, Second Edition:
Helping Patients Change Behavior
Stephen Rollnick, William R. Miller, and Christopher C. Butler

Motivational Interviewing, Fourth Edition:
Helping People Change and Grow
William R. Miller and Stephen Rollnick

Motivational Interviewing in Life and Health Coaching:
A Guide to Effective Practice
Cecilia H. Lanier, Patty Bean, and Stacey C. Arnold

Motivational Interviewing across Cultures:
Optimizing Practice
Christina S. Lee

Motivational Interviewing in the Treatment
of Psychological Problems, Third Edition
Brian L. Burke, Brad Lundahl, and Hal Arkowitz, Editors

Motivational Interviewing with Families
Douglas C. Smith

Motivational Interviewing in Nutrition and Fitness,
Second Edition
Dawn Clifford and Laura Curtis

MOTIVATIONAL INTERVIEWING WITH FAMILIES

Douglas C. Smith

*Series Editors' Note by William R. Miller,
Theresa B. Moyers, and Stephen Rollnick*

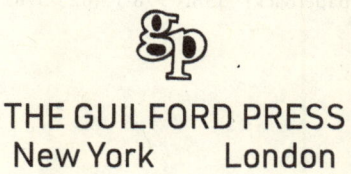

THE GUILFORD PRESS
New York   London

Copyright © 2025 The Guilford Press
A Division of Guilford Publications, Inc.
www.guilford.com

All rights reserved

No part of this book may be reproduced, translated, stored in a retrieval system, or transmitted, in any form or by any means, electronic, mechanical, photocopying, microfilming, recording, or otherwise, without written permission from the publisher.

Printed in the United States of America

This book is printed on acid-free paper.

For product and safety concerns within the EU, please contact GPSR@taylorandfrancis.com, Taylor & Francis Verlag GmbH, Kaufingerstraße 24, 80331 München, Germany.

Last digit is print number: 9 8 7 6 5 4 3 2 1

The author has checked with sources believed to be reliable in his efforts to provide information that is complete and generally in accord with the standards of practice that are accepted at the time of publication. However, in view of the possibility of human error or changes in behavioral, mental health, or medical sciences, neither the author, nor the editor and publisher, nor any other party who has been involved in the preparation or publication of this work warrants that the information contained herein is in every respect accurate or complete, and they are not responsible for any errors or omissions or the results obtained from the use of such information. Readers are encouraged to confirm the information contained in this book with other sources.

Library of Congress Cataloging-in-Publication Data is available from the publisher.

ISBN 978-1-4625-5761-5 (paperback)   ISBN 978-1-4625-5762-2 (hardcover)

To Carol

About the Author

Douglas C. Smith, PhD, LCSW, is Professor of Social Work at the University of Illinois at Urbana–Champaign. He is a member of the Motivational Interviewing Network of Trainers (MINT) and co-chair of MINT's Professional Development Committee. Dr. Smith is a recipient of the Deborah K. Padgett Early Career Achievement Award from the Society for Social Work and Research. His research and publications focus on motivational interviewing and on developing and testing substance use interventions—including family therapies—for adolescents and emerging adults.

Series Editors' Note

There are very good reasons to be working with families. Although the history of psychotherapy has focused primarily on counseling individuals, family members are intimately involved with each other's well-being and suffering. They usually care about and want to help each other and may play an important role in the concerns being addressed in treatment. Intimate loved ones usually know more about us than anyone else does, sometimes more than we know about ourselves. Family members are *involved* in outcomes and can provide vital support for each other. Furthermore, there is clear research evidence that treatment outcomes are often better when concerned partners, parents, or significant others are involved in the process.

We are particularly pleased, therefore, to have this addition to Guilford's Applications of Motivational Interviewing series. This has been an important missing piece, and Doug Smith has done a masterful job of conveying how motivational interviewing (MI) is effectively practiced with two or more related people. In this volume, he has drawn together clinical science, seasoned experience, and practical wisdom. He makes a persuasive case that the compassionate, accepting, partnering, and empowering approach of MI is particularly well suited for helping families change and grow.

MI is closely attuned to language. What clients say during treatment sessions influences their outcomes and is in turn affected by clinical skills that are clarified in MI. Working with families adds a level of complexity because clients also influence each other's speech. Smith takes MI to this next level of interpersonal skill and introduces the concept of family-level change talk.

For clinicians who have been using MI with individuals, *Motivational Interviewing with Families* will help extend your work and practice to couples and families in their many modern configurations. After all, families are those who care for and support each other, not necessarily defined by bloodlines or legal arrangements. For counselors already accustomed to working with families, Doug Smith amply illustrates how MI can render your work more rewarding and effective, explaining how the spirit and practical skills of MI can be integrated to enrich family-centered care. And for those interested in family processes, he adds a rich layer of linguistic complexity to motivation for change and growth.

May you find in this volume new insights to inform your clinical work and ultimately to benefit the families whom you serve.

WILLIAM R. MILLER, PhD
THERESA B. MOYERS, PhD
STEPHEN ROLLNICK, PhD

Preface

Although various adaptations of motivational interviewing (MI) have included family members, very limited theoretical work exists to guide us on how to use MI when more than one person is sitting in the consultation room. I found that curious because my work has involved family members and friendship dyads. People in our clients' social networks matter tremendously, and working with them may help improve our clients' outcomes. This book represents the culmination of 20 years of work in applying MI in my practice with families and dyads.

This book is both theoretical and practical. As a student, I always enjoyed reading material that included concrete examples of how to do interventions. Nothing frustrated me more than learning about an empirically supported intervention in the abstract. That is, I heard a lot about interventions I should be doing through lecture material, but nobody showed me how to do them!

Later on as a teacher, I developed a course on MI where master's-level social work (MSW) students' key assignments involved submitting audio recordings of their MI practice. It was one of the most skill-intensive courses we offered before students entered their internships. They learned the theory of MI through practicing the skills interactively.

I've brought this practical perspective to this book. Although I introduced some new definitions and could not shy away from theory, I didn't want to lose sight of creating a practical book. I hope that the following pages provide you with ample opportunities to see what MI looks like when used with families. Additionally, I hope the exercises throughout the book deepen your understanding of MI. I wish you luck on your journey toward integrating MI into your important work with families.

A few notes about the content and language used in this book bear mentioning. First, the case material used in this book is both fictional and real. None of the case material uses direct quotes from actual therapy sessions. When examples draw on real cases, extensive efforts were made to prevent the identification of former clients. Second, I have defined family broadly to include families we are born into and those we select. Defining what constitutes a family is tricky, and most health professionals recognize substantial diversity among families. A similar challenge in writing this book involved using gender-neutral language. I tried to avoid using gendered pronouns whenever possible, except when to do so would create clarity issues in case examples. Finally, throughout the book, I refer to the health professional who uses MI as "helper." However, I use the terms "client" and "patient" and "family member" interchangeably to refer to people seeking services. Some fields have their preferred language conventions for this. As I was writing to a broad clinical audience, this mix of terms was intended only to capture this diversity.

Acknowledgments

I would like thank Jim Nageotte and Jane Keislar at The Guilford Press for their endless patience with me. The writing of this book was interrupted by a global pandemic and the loss of my father. Without their nonstop encouragement and keen editing skills, this book would not have come to fruition. Series Editor Dr. William Miller was also inspirational in helping me find my voice at a time when I was floundering.

I'd like to thank all the members of the Motivational Interviewing Network of Trainers' Professional Development Committee (MINT PDC). Your encouragement has meant a lot to me. Special thanks to the committee co-chair, Dr. Kate Speck, for reading early drafts of the manuscript. Special thanks also go out to MINT PDC committee member Dr. Heloísa Garcia Claro Fernandes, for helping me develop training materials based on this book for use with Brazilian families.

I'd like to also thank the wonderful staff at the Youth Services Network in Rockford, Illinois, for providing me with feedback on early training materials based on this book. Your work with families in crisis inspired me when my motivation to finish this book was ebbing. For that you have my thanks.

Contents

PART I. THE BASICS

1. Introduction	3
2. Overview of Motivational Interviewing	15
3. The Spirit of Motivational Interviewing	24
4. ROARS Skills	39
5. Working with Ambivalence	54

PART II. USING MOTIVATIONAL INTERVIEWING WITH FAMILIES

6. Moving toward Integration of Motivational Interviewing and Family Work	75
7. Advanced Issues in Using ROARS with Families	91
8. Change Talk among Families	100
9. Engaging Families with Motivational Interviewing	121

10. Focusing, Evoking, and Planning in Family Work	142
11. Motivational Sendoffs	154

PART III. FAMILY-CENTERED MOTIVATIONAL INTERVIEWING RESEARCH

12. Families Raising and Launching Children with Alex Lee	167
13. Families with Established and Older Adults	188
APPENDIX. Select Resources for Integrating Motivational Interviewing in Family Work	203
References	209
Index	231

> Purchasers of this book can access clickable links
> to the resources described in the Appendix
> at *www.guilford.com/smith10-materials*.

PART I
THE BASICS

CHAPTER 1

Introduction

> No man is an island.
> —JOHN DONNE

Whether one's closest social ties are to blood relatives or to individuals not biologically related, everyone belongs to a family. Families morph, adding and subtracting members across the life cycle. Family configurations also vary widely in modern society (Roseneil & Budgeon, 2004; Walsh, 2012), and the importance and meaning of family varies across cultures. Nevertheless, few people would deny belonging to a family.

Families maintain a central role in educating, socializing, caring for, emotionally supporting, and healing their members. Briar-Lawson and colleagues (2001) described families as "comprehensive social welfare institutions" that have more responsibilities for their members than any social or health service providers could ever possibly have. For example, with arguably few exceptions, families never get to discharge their members.[1]

The primacy of the family, in whatever shape it may take, cannot be underestimated. For example, vast health benefits exist for maintaining close family ties. Married individuals live longer, and engage in less risky

---

[1] In the United States, all 50 states have "safe haven" laws where desperate parents who believe they cannot care for their child can cede their child to the State's care (Child Welfare Information Gateway, 2017). These laws are intended to save infants' lives based on estimates of deaths of unwanted children (Herman-Giddens et al., 2003). I could not locate a credible national estimate of abandoned babies, but some research suggests that the rate is fairly low, with 1,479 total babies surrendered nationally from 1999 to 2008 (Porter, 2010).

behavior, than unmarried people (Waite, 1985, Wang et al., 2020). Parenting and family communication buffer against a number of adolescent and young adult problems, such as substance use (Hawkins et al., 1992), delinquency (Hoeve et al., 2009), obesity (Dallacker et al., 2019; Pinquart, 2014), and leaving school before graduating (Strom & Boster, 2007). Family dissolution due to divorce is recognized as an adverse childhood experience and negatively impacts children if not handled well. Families care for children and adult members with disabilities. Later in the lifespan, millions of family members provide caregiving to their elders, allowing them to age in place (Schulz et al., 2020). It is no wonder that numerous social policies are designed with families in mind, including adoption, taxation, child support, and family leave benefits.

Why, then, do the helping professions and clinical scientists focus primarily on providing services only to individuals? For example, there are twice as many systematic reviews on person-centered versus family-centered health care (Park et al., 2018). This suggests that there exist barriers to implementing family-centered care. Such barriers could include lack of insurance reimbursement for family-centered care (Clawson et al., 2018; Tambling et al., 2020), an inadequately prepared workforce (Goodyear et al., 2017), family members deciding not to engage in services due to family conflict or fear of being scapegoated, and perceptions from clients that family-based intervention is not needed or won't work (McPherson et al., 2017).

WHAT IS "FAMILY" AND "FAMILY-CENTERED CARE"?

In this book **family** is defined as a group of two or more people that regularly provide support to one another, regardless of shared bloodlines or legal arrangements (Holtzman, 2008). Indeed, families presenting to helping professionals take on myriad configurations, including the following: gay, lesbian, transgender, or heteronormative couples who are or are not legally married; parent–child or grandparent–child dyads; a friendship dyad; a long-term mentor and a child in state custody who resides in a group home; or biological parents and their children. This list is clearly not exhaustive (see the box on page 5).

I define **family-centered care** here as any professional or paraprofessional service in which more than one member of a family sees the same helper. Importantly, family members could visit the same helper together at the same time or in separate consultations. Thus, family-centered care is not limited to family therapy or services

The principles of family-centered care are consistent with the spirit of MI.

> **My Journey of Integrating MI with Family-Centered Care**
>
> Early in my career, I was a clinical supervisor of a small adolescent substance use treatment unit. When I started, no family services existed, despite really promising research support for it. Teens met individually with counselors or in groups with other teens. Back then, rallying cries existed for providing more family services. One highly influential paper suggested that providing group therapy to teens could actually make their problems worse because they'd negatively influence each other (Dishion et al., 1999).
>
> When adding family services, we required that one family member attend the teen's initial substance use assessment. We were concerned that families would not attend. I had heard about MI and had received some initial training. To integrate families, but also respect teen autonomy, we developed a family-centered assessment debriefing session where we first met with the teen, then met privately with the parent, and finally met conjointly (Smith & Hall, 2007). MI was used with both parents and teens in hopes that it would help engage them into treatment. It worked, especially for teens who didn't initially think they had problems with substances (Smith et al., 2009).
>
> Because of my positive experiences with engaging families with MI, I ultimately joined the Motivational Interviewing Network of Trainers (MINT; see Appendix). MINT is an international group of MI trainers who want to provide high-quality training and prevent the spread of misinformation about the use of MI. I've more recently been using MI in work with young adult friendship dyads, which I consider "selected families."
>
> **THOUGHT QUESTIONS:** (1) What motivates you to learn about family-centered care? (2) What are some challenges in providing family-centered care? (3) In your own words, how do you define "family"?

provided by graduates of an accredited marriage and family therapy program. The principles of family-centered care (Bamm et al., 2008), such as recognizing families as strong and unique entities, or engaging families as equal partners in health decisions, are consistent with the spirit with which motivational interviewing (MI) is delivered.

Families often seek care when they have concerns about one of their members. This member will be referred to as the **identified client**. The quintessential identified client is a person with a severe substance use problem receiving a family intervention. In interventions, each member tells the identified client how their behavior is affecting them, encourages the identified client to seek treatment, and gives ultimatums should future substance use occur. Many people are familiar with family interventions through the popular media. For example, the A&E television show titled *Intervention* showed families providing interventions to loved ones with severe addictions (Kosovski & Smith, 2011). In short, family-centered care sometimes involves recognizing whether the family is seeking treatment due to an identified client's behavior.

Family-centered care exists in several settings. Examples include family psychoeducational groups occurring in residential treatment, case management services provided during elder protection services, primary care appointments where family members are present, and psychiatric services that involve sporadic family involvement during appointments. Because the backgrounds of those providing family-centered care vary widely, I will use the term **helper** throughout this book to refer to the person in the role of providing care. This term is meant to be inclusive, as many professionals work with families, but would not define their work as family therapy.

EFFICACY OF FAMILY MODELS

Voluminous empirical support exists for family-centered interventions. Such interventions are efficacious for adolescent suicidal ideation (Waraan et al., 2023), youth with disruptive behavior problems (Sheidow et al., 2022), substance use disorders (Ariss & Fairbairn, 2020), marital distress (Wood et al., 2005), pediatric obesity treatment (Janicke et al., 2014), and mental health services (Barbato & D'Avanzo, 2008; Riedinger et al., 2017). Although more research is needed, family-centered interventions even show promise in select situations where intimate partner violence occurs (Karakurt et al., 2016). This finding surprised some clinical researchers that were initially reluctant to use family therapies with families experiencing violence, to the point that some studies excluded such families. There is little doubt that family-centered services, if implemented well, can ameliorate a number of health and psychosocial problems.

Potential Mechanisms of Change

What factors account for the success of family-centered care? Clinical science has started moving past the question of what treatments work for most people. This relatively simple question is answered by studying whether a treatment, on average, works for families receiving it. Yet, there are no average families, and treatment responses vary. Thus, we now concern ourselves with not only knowing what works, but also for whom and why. Understanding why a treatment works is commonly referred to as the mechanism of change. A mechanism of change is a process through which a treatment produces its effect.

Several potential mechanisms of change may operate in family-centered care. First, increasing multiple family members' knowledge about a particular problem is empowering. This is commonly referred to as family psychoeducation, which is important and highly effective for some presenting problems, especially for mental health treatment (Lyman et al., 2014). Second, it may reduce family conflict, which often provokes the presenting problem in the first place. Consider that marital discord is clearly associated with several childhood behavior problems (Reid & Crisafulli, 1990), depression and inflammation (Kiecolt-Glaser, 2018), and likely a host of other reasons families seek care. Treating relational discord and increasing family problem-solving skills among families may produce salubrious effects. For example, increases in family problem-solving skills are longitudinally linked to improvements in diabetes (Wysocki et al., 2008). Finally, family-centered care may also be beneficial because of the ability of family members to check up on each other and hold each other accountable outside of therapy sessions. Perhaps this is why some family-centered care models produce more durable effects than individually based treatments (Liddle et al., 2008).

CHALLENGES IN FAMILY-CENTERED CARE

Although family-centered care is efficacious, helpers often encounter two key challenges. First, families often discontinue care earlier than recommended. Additionally, helpers must hone their communications skills to develop strong therapeutic alliances with families. These two challenges are interrelated. That is, weak alliances are related to premature exits from family-centered care.

Choosing to Leave Care

Often, family members do not engage in treatment. Also, sometimes they choose to leave before receiving enough of a therapeutic dose.[2] For exam-

---

[2] I refrain from using the term "dropout," especially in reference to family members. Instead, I will use more neutral and person-first terms like "when services end abruptly" or "families who chose to end services." Framing early exits from treatment as "dropout" is inconsistent with the humanizing spirit of MI and emphasis on family members' autonomy.

ple, many people are familiar with the concept of a family intervention when one member suffers from an addiction. As mentioned earlier, in this model, family members confront a loved one with an addiction in an effort to get them into treatment (Kosovksi & Smith, 2011). Although interventions work at engaging loved ones in treatment, one study found that as few as 30% of families completed the intervention (Miller et al., 1999). Widespread implementation of a treatment that 70% of families ultimately choose not to do is difficult to justify. Such a treatment would not reach enough people. Despite their continuing popularity in the mainstream media, little recent research exists on such interventions.

Electing to leave family-centered care early is a common occurrence. Even when families have resources such as good health care insurance, almost one in five clients seeing a trained marriage and family therapist did not return for a second session (Hamilton et al., 2011). This rate may be an underestimate, too, as other studies suggest rates between 20 and 50%, likely depending on the characteristics of families, providers, and settings (Cooper et al., 2018). Hamilton and colleagues (2011) also showed that family therapy clients were 33.2% more likely to leave treatment prematurely compared with clients receiving individual therapy.

Helpers providing family-centered care must grapple with the problem of families not wanting to engage or remain in treatment. McAdams and colleagues' (2018) systematic review identified six actionable strategies to boost family therapy retention, including (1) conveying understanding and support, (2) demonstrating knowledge and support, (3) communicating a genuine desire to help, (4) clearly describing the family therapy process, (5) communicating hope that problems can be resolved, and (6) creating a safe environment. As you will see in later chapters, several of these strategies are consistent with the approach presented in this book, MI. I wrote this book in hopes of introducing this model to helpers who want to increase family engagement.

The transtheoretical model of behavioral change, commonly known as the stages-of-change model, offers a perspective on why families may choose to leave care early (Prochaska et al., 1992) The model suggests that family members may vary on their readiness to make behavioral changes. The theory posits several different stages, including precontemplation, contemplation, preparation, action, and maintenance. Precontemplation involves limited awareness or belief that change is needed. Contemplation, as the moniker suggests, occurs when family members are thinking about whether or not they need to change. Family members in the preparation stage acknowledge the need for change but have not actively started on a plan of action. Those in the action stage have done just that. Finally, those in maintenance, as the label suggests, have made some changes and work to sustain them.

Limited research exists on the stages-of-change model and retention in family-centered care. One early study by Tambling and Johnson (2008) found that a couple's stage of change did not predict retention or outcomes. Also, men scored lower than women on motivation for change. However, the findings from this early study may have been due to inadequate measurement of the stages of change. That is, in a subsequent study that used a measure of stages of change specific to relationships (i.e., Relational Version of the University of Rhode Island Change Assessment [R-URICA]; Tambling & Ketring, 2014), stage of change did predict outcomes (Tambling & Johnson, 2019). In short, the stages-of-change model seems to be a viable heuristic for thinking about families' readiness to change.

On Therapeutic Alliances

Therapeutic alliances refer to family members' feeling a strong bond to the helper and agreement on what goals will be addressed. Therapeutic alliance is related to both treatment retention and outcomes (Anderson et al., 2019; Del Re et. al., 2021; Friedlander et al., 2018).

An important point is that, no matter what evidence-based practice model a helper uses, they should invest in developing strong communication skills. For example, one recent meta-analysis shows that helpers have varying degrees of skill in developing therapeutic alliances (Del Re et al., 2021). Thus, in addition to developing expertise in clinical methods, helpers should also focus on their communication skills (see the box on page 10).

So, what may be some important dimensions of therapeutic alliances that may be honed by learning MI? Research shows that working on engagement, being able to provide a safe environment, and collaboratively setting goals are critical skills. For example, Sotero and Relvas (2021) reviewed video tapes of 40 family therapy sessions and examined associations between four different dimensions of therapeutic alliance and retention in treatment. Dimensions included engagement, safety, emotional connection, and a shared sense of purpose. They found that engagement, safety, and shared sense of purpose were all higher among retained cases.

Potential Benefits of Learning MI

So much has been written on families leaving care and therapeutic alliance that it is beyond the scope of this book to cover each comprehensively.

However, the point is that MI can strengthen therapeutic alliances and increase retention in family-centered care. Focusing on familial motivation for change would be beneficial. Many families elect to discontinue treatment due to low motivation (D'Aniello et al., 2019). Thus, helpers need to be able to identify families that may be at risk for premature termination of services. Additionally, they should develop skills that effectively engage and retain clients. Throughout this book, I will present concrete examples of how to engage family members reluctant to attend sessions, address how to negotiate goals with high levels of collaboration (i.e., a key aspect of therapeutic alliance), and use other communication skills that may ultimately strengthen alliances.

MI can increase retention in family-centered care.

The Importance of Learning Communication Skills

I once did a training with a community organization tasked with responding to family crises that may result in detention or the need to secure emergency housing for teens. We role-played one such crisis, which involved empathizing with both parental and teen perceptions of family conflict. After the role playing, one of the participants commented on how using the skills in the demonstration could potentially shorten their interactions with families.

Helpers develop certain communication strategies with families, which sometimes are less direct and inefficient. My interpretation of this trainee comment is that there is a persistent need for developing communication skills to build familial motivation. MI is one tool for rapidly developing therapeutic alliances in even the most difficult scenarios. These trainees had substantial expertise in common familial disputes, yet found something new in MI that could benefit their work.

This brings us to a key point. MI is a conversational style to be used in concert with whatever family-centered care model one uses. It is not intended to be a comprehensive family-centered care model. Instead, it may aid helpers in doing the family work they do better. It can help address key challenges in family work through teaching communication skills and a way of being with families.

THOUGHT QUESTIONS: (1) Which of your communication skills do you use well? (2) Which of your communications skills could use improvement? (3) How do you know when you are communicating effectively?

A Taste of MI

MI involves compassionate conversations about change. It is particularly useful for resolving ambivalence about change and assumes that such ambivalence about change is a natural part of the change process. It refrains from pathologizing such reluctance to change. That is, instead of labeling families as "dropouts," "hard to treat," or "resistant," as if these are intrinsic traits, helpers using MI seek to gain an in-depth understanding of their families' motivations. They work to resolve ambivalence about change. Some helpers like to think of MI as a way to guide families though the aforementioned stages of change.

Rather than prescriptively identifying solutions for families, MI seeks to empower families to solve their own problems. Family members are active collaborators in the change process, rather than passive recipients of the helper's wisdom. In other words, this approach achieves much better buy-in from families.

MI is based on Rogerian therapy and has been refined over the past 40 years through numerous process studies where scientists listened carefully to conversations about change. Through this research, clinical scientists have identified what they think are some of the active ingredients that make MI work.

What is particularly stunning about this work is that it turns out that what helpers say impacts what clients say during sessions. It also turns out that what we sometimes label resistance may not be an intrinsic trait of families at all. Instead, it may be a byproduct of how helpers talk to family members. For example, a well-intentioned helper may inadvertently increase a family member's resistance or ambivalence about change. This happens right in front of our very eyes because what clients say during sessions predicts actual change. Thus, part of using MI in family-centered care involves deep listening to family members' statements about change.

> **MI involves deep listening to family members' statements about change.**

At this writing, there exist only a few efforts to integrate MI in family-centered care, most of which are limited to the substance use disorder[3] field. This book seeks to introduce MI to helpers providing a wider range of family-centered services so that additional integration efforts will occur.

---

[3] Many readers may be accustomed to the term "substance abuse treatment." However, data show that the term "substance abuse" increases stigma (Kelly & Westerhoff, 2010; Kelly et al., 2021).

OPPORTUNITIES FOR USING MI IN FAMILY-CENTERED CARE

Multiple opportunities exist for using MI in family-centered care. Here, I review some common dilemmas in work with families where MI may prove useful:

Scenario 1

A child protection worker meets with two parents who have just lost their children to the child protection system. The task is to communicate the court's expectations for them if they pursue family reunification. There are many requirements, such as obtaining employment, attending all court hearings, increasing home safety, attending parenting classes, and reducing substance use. Families in this situation frequently get angry with their caseworkers. Such families interacting with multiple social service systems often do not trust workers in these systems. It is common for them to miss appointments. The worker is looking for a counseling method where they can treat all families with dignity, motivate families, and communicate the requirements of the court.

Scenario 2

A helper is approached by a 45-year-old woman about relational trouble she has been having with her partner. Her partner exhibits signs of depression, and they have numerous arguments. They have been in a committed relationship for over a decade, but she said she felt they have gradually become more distant the past couple of years. She'd like to try couples counseling but is not sure if her partner will be willing to join her in that venture. She thinks her partner will be defensive and feel singled out. The helper is looking for an effective way to engage with the partner.

Scenario 3

A teenager involved in the criminal legal system is in constant conflict with their parents. The helper worked with them on coping strategies and communication skills that the teen can implement, which led to some improvements. However, frequent fighting continues unabated, and the teen feels that their parents' love is conditional. The helper proposed involving the parents in some sessions. The teen, however, voices some reluctance. The helper wishes there was a way to broach the subject again but doesn't want to alienate the teenager.

Scenario 4

A caseworker made a plan with an elderly woman and her middle-aged son to transition her from in-home care to living in an assisted living community. Yet, when the helper met with them again, the woman and her son did not complete any of their tasks. The helper recognizes the need to reevaluate whether their goals have changed. Their professional opinion is that conditions at the home are becoming increasingly unsafe, with elevated risks for falling, failing to take medications, and eating inconsistently. The helper feels like they have lost some momentum and wants to revisit the action plan.

MY HOPE FOR THIS BOOK

This book introduces MI (Miller & Rollnick, 2023) to helpers providing family-centered care. It assumes limited knowledge of MI and is meant to help providers integrate it into their work with families. Most of my professional experience using MI involves integrating it into family therapy with adolescents, as well as with friendship dyads. However, I've written this book in a manner in which it can be used whether or not readers are providing family therapy proper. All providers, whether they provide bona fide family therapy or not, will encounter a critical problem in family-centered care, the need to effectively engage families and work with those who appear reluctant to change. This book addresses the problem of motivating a wide range of families across multiple health and social services settings.

I don't present a single, overarching therapy program that integrates MI and a specific family therapy model. However, Chapter 6 reviews various family therapy models and their compatibility with MI. Instead, this book will identify multiple opportunities for using MI, no matter how you want to work with families. I argue that MI could be one plausible strategy for engaging and retaining family members in care. Like any therapy model, MI will not be a panacea for all your families' problems (Miller & Rollnick, 2009). Yet, MI can provide helpers with a framework for thinking about motivation, as well as concrete tools to address common impasses.

SUMMARY

Family-centered care is efficacious for a wide range of psychosocial problems. Yet, helpers vary widely in their communication skills, which affect therapeutic alliances. This in turn leads to families deciding to exit services prematurely, before achieving maximum benefits. MI is a conversational style that can aid helpers in their family work. In Chapter 2, I will define MI and begin discussing how these communication skills can aid family work.

CHAPTER 2

Overview of Motivational Interviewing

> Learning to conduct a motivational interview isn't easy. It involves . . . principles of dyadic communication, some of which are explicitly delineated as "skills" while others are acquired more osmotically as "spirit" . . . clients will feel more befriended than bossed into behavior change.
> —E. SUMMERSON CARR

In Chapter 1, I discussed how MI may be helpful in various family-centered care contexts. In this chapter, I provide a brief history of the development of MI. Then, I expand on the core elements of MI. Finally, I apply the principles of MI to a case example involving family work to illustrate its application.

A BRIEF HISTORY OF MI

Dr. William R. Miller, Professor Emeritus of Psychology at the University of New Mexico, initially formulated MI (Miller, 1983). At the time, individuals with substance use disorders were frequently characterized as pathological liars, personality-disordered, and generally lacking insight about their maladies. Moralistic models of substance use drove this conceptualization, which viewed individuals with substance use disorders as morally flawed. Confrontational approaches designed to break through denial ran rampant in that era.

Research, however, started revealing that the more you confronted individuals with substance use problems, the more they drank (Miller et al., 1993). So, a conundrum existed: If confrontation was so good at promoting self-awareness among individuals in denial, why did they drink more? It did not add up. Miller's early discoveries were followed up with a major clinical trial that established MI as an evidence-based treatment for alcohol use disorders (Project MATCH Research Group, 1998). MI was found to have equivalent outcomes as cognitive-behavioral therapy (CBT) and twelve-step facilitation therapy (TSF). Research on MI in the addictions field began to flourish.

Apparently, the substance use disorder (SUD) field did not have a monopoly on addressing ambivalence about change. That is, MI began to take off in areas of health care outside of the addictions field. To date, there are over 2,000 controlled trials on MI, and nearly 200 systematic reviews and meta-analyses (Miller & Rollnick, 2023). Meta-analyses are aggregate studies of clinical trials that examine the impact of MI across all studies that meet pre-specified inclusion criteria. For example, some meta-analyses focus on a specific population, such as one my colleagues and I did on the effectiveness of substance use treatments for non-college-attending young adults (Davis et al., 2017). Mine and other meta-analyses generally report positive findings for MI relative to control conditions (Borrelli et al., 2015; Hettema et al., 2005; Lundahl et al., 2010; Rubak et al., 2005).

Because MI is so firmly established, efforts now focus on determining how MI works, how to best train helpers to learn it, and how to adapt it to new contexts such as family work. I hope that one day there is enough research on using MI with families that a meta-analysis may be done. There is little research on using MI in family-centered care contexts, which I will summarize in later chapters.

WHAT IS MI?

In a nutshell, MI is an approach to having a compassionate conversation designed to reduce client ambivalence about change. Rather than conceptualizing individuals as resistant, lacking insight, or being in denial when they express disinterest in change, MI sees ambivalence as the normal push–pull process of change. That is, individuals, and here families, may have a litany of reasons for not making a particular change.

MI sees ambivalence as normal.

Resolving Ambivalence

Behavior change is hard. This may be especially true for making emotionally charged changes that involve one's family. Consider some examples of ambivalence that we may see in family work:

- An elder who is reluctant to set boundaries with her grown daughter who recently moved into her house following a divorce.
- A single mother who questions whether involvement in her child's treatment will matter. The parent tells you, "He's grown and has to make his own choices."
- One member of a couple who does not want to attend couples counseling.
- A caregiver who does not want to make diet changes, or monitor his child's food choices, to help his child reduce his weight.

MI assumes that, if helpers push too hard for change before a client has resolved their ambivalence, families will naturally push back. Importantly, this is not resistance per se, but rather voicing naturally occurring reservations about the costs of change. So, just as laws of physics suggest that objects impacted by some force will naturally counteract with force, so it goes with our ambivalent clients. Rather than provoking such a collision of the wills, MI seeks to resolve such ambivalence using alternative strategies besides cajoling, convincing, persuading, or confronting. In fact, this compassionate method seeks to induce clients into talking themselves into change.

Three Core Elements of MI

The three core elements of MI are (1) an underlying spirit that emphasizes partnership, acceptance, compassion, and empowerment; (2) masterful use of micro-counseling skills; and (3) emphasis on identifying and reinforcing client change talk. Let us describe each of these three components in detail here.

MI Spirit

Partnership, acceptance, compassion, and empowerment comprise the four key components of the MI Spirit (Miller & Rollnick, 2023). Partnership involves sharing power with families and actively seeking and using their expertise in the development of solutions. Acceptance involves taking a nonjudgmental perspective on the family as they are, period. Compassion refers to holding the family's interests at the center of the helping relationship. Finally, empowerment deals with building both decision-making and other problem-solving skills while enhancing the family's sense that they can effect change. Chapter 3 elaborates on all these components of the MI Spirit.

Micro-Counseling Skills

The four main skills used in MI form the handy acronym OARS. They include open questions, affirmations, reflections, and summaries.[1] Many helpers possess familiarity with these skills, so I only provide brief coverage here and focus more on the theory-driven manner in which they are used in MI in the next section on change talk. In my opinion, beginning learners may know the structure of many of these statements but need guidance in how to use them strategically. Importantly, what separates MI from generalist use of OARS rests in a data-driven approach to learning which combinations have a better chance at getting to change.

Regarding questions, open ones typically beckon longer, thoughtful replies from clients. Closed questions, by contrast, are those that usually generate short replies or specific information. Affirmations are positive statements about a family's traits or efforts. Reflections are statements that reword client content and can either be very simple restatements (e.g., you're sad) or increasingly vivid and complex (e.g., this is like having your teeth pulled without anesthesia). Finally, summaries are basically just long reflections that capture much more session content. I dedicate all of Chapter 4 to defining and illustrating the use of these skills.

Change Talk and Sustain Talk

Listening deeply to what clients say is a longstanding and research-informed aspect of MI (Amhrein et al., 2003; Magill et al., 2018). Simply stated, the main goal of MI is to resolve ambivalence by evoking and reinforcing change talk within a compassionate environment.

Change talk is formally defined as any client speech in the direction of change. It is yoked to a particular target behavior, is usually in the here and now, and can be elicited deliberately using the OARS skills. Evoking means calling out motivation that is already there instead of telling families why or how they should change. Once families give voice to change talk, helpers using MI try to deepen the conversation about it by reflecting, asking for more details, affirming, or summarizing it.

> **Evoking means calling out motivation that is already there.**

Sustain talk, however, is language in favor of the status quo. Again, sustain talk is considered a normal part of the change process and not

---

[1] In Chapter 4, I advocate for changing this acronym to ROARS, because of the central role of reflections in MI. ROARS stands for reflections, open questions, affirmations, and reflective summaries.

indicative of denial, obstinacy, lack of motivation, or resistance. In fact, sometimes sustain talk is inevitable, so helpers using MI are trained to empathize with sustain talk, softening its impact. It is often important to acknowledge, but now wallow in, sustain talk.

Empathically shifting conversations from sustain talk and toward change talk requires masterful and strategic use of OARS skills. For example, helpers can inadvertently say things that are more likely to elicit sustain talk, even if their efforts were well intentioned. Although it may be forgivable for a hard play in sports to result in an error, a routine play resulting in an error is sometimes called an "unforced" error. Avoiding unforced errors in MI would involve refraining from saying things that elicit client sustain talk. Consider the open question, "How do you feel about doing this?" It is so open that a client could respond with either change talk, sustain talk, or a mixture of both. In one study, open questions were followed by sustain talk about 20% of the time (Apodaca et al., 2016). I think this has to do with each question's specific nature; not all open questions are created equal. Some are better for probing change talk than others.

Another unforced error would involve using persuasion or confrontation with family members. MI doesn't involve using either of these tactics. Research shows that using confrontation has a higher probability of being followed by sustain talk (Gaume et al., 2008; Apodaca et al., 2016). Furthermore, it is normal for family members, unprovoked by the helper, to voice sustain talk. In this situation, there is sometimes a temptation for helpers to argue against it via confrontation or persuasion. However, this also is hypothesized to result in clients digging in and standing their ground.

Equipoise occurs when a clinician explicitly decides not to privilege change talk. Specifically, equipoise refers to maintaining neutrality with regards to evoking the language of change. So, equipoise is about deliberately avoiding one core feature of MI where clinicians use OARS skills strategically to resolve ambivalence in the direction of a particular change (i.e., target behavior). There are sometimes ethical reasons for doing this. In family work, as we will discuss in later chapters, there are also several nuances regarding how you reinforce change language for one family member while not alienating another in conjoint sessions. We will deal with these types of advanced challenges in Chapter 8.

A BRIEF CASE EXAMPLE

Here, I demonstrate the difference between two contrasting clinical approaches. The first example does not use MI; the second one does. In both examples, a helper wants to encourage a teenager to add family sessions to what is currently individual therapy. The only difference in the two examples is how the helper goes about communicating this idea.

Example 1: Encouraging a Family Session without MI

HELPER: You know, we really should consider bringing your parents in for a session.

CLIENT: I don't know. They'd probably just fight in front of you.

HELPER: I hear you. But do you know that research shows that family therapy can really help. It is really successful with other teens who have had the same problem. [A persuasion attempt]

CLIENT: But this is my family we are talking about. I can barely deal with my own shit. I don't want a stressful session with them.

HELPER: Aw, come on. It can't be that bad. Besides, when I see them here, we can tell them how you feel about their fighting, and that may make things better for you at home. [Another persuasion attempt]

Here, the helper expresses their firm belief that family involvement will help this teen, which research supports. Yet, the teen responds to the helpers' initial suggestion with ambivalence, expressing concerns about what that would look like. As noted above, this is exactly what MI is useful in addressing. However, instead of using OARS skills to soften this ambivalence and steer the conversation to a more productive place, the helper meets the ambivalence by presenting the teen with research information and their own practice wisdom. This is an example of taking an **expert stance** instead of enhancing partnership. An expert stance involves a helper saying they know what is best for their clients, and sometimes doubling down when they encounter pushback. Thus, the helper does not elicit change talk about any of the potential benefits that may exist for the client if a family session occurred.

Example 2: Encouraging a Family Session Using MI

So, what would this same conversation look like if the helper used MI? Below, in a very short exchange, I will illustrate all three components of the MI intervention, including the use of the MI spirit, the OARS skills, and the emphasis on generating client language in favor of change.

HELPER: I've had an idea I've been toying around with, and I'm curious if you'd like to hear it. [Enhancing autonomy]

CLIENT: Go ahead.

HELPER: So, it's up to you if we do this or not. I've been wondering if it may help to have your parents attend a session. This has been helpful with other clients facing problems similar to yours. What are your thoughts on that? [Enhancing autonomy and collaboration]

CLIENT: I don't know. They'd probably just fight in front of you.

HELPER: And that would be painful and embarrassing for you to watch. [Reflection, empathic, focused on sustain talk]

CLIENT: Yep. Cringe-worthy.

HELPER: Ah, so you could really see that backfiring and are pretty sure that nothing good would come out of it. [Reflection, empathic, change talk]

CLIENT: I don't know. It may help me if you backed me up when I tell them some things I've been meaning to get off my chest.

HELPER: So, it may be worth risking, if you could get me in your corner for some things. And it would help you to get some things off your chest. [Reflection, highlighting change talk]

CLIENT: Yeah, but it would also be difficult.

HELPER: You need to think through whether it is worth it. I'll support you no matter what you decide. [Reflection, highlighting empathy and autonomy]

So, what was different here? The client was the same, having the same mixed feelings about parental intrusion (i.e., fear of devolving into parental fighting, potential embarrassment). However, here the helper asked permission to make a suggestion, which is thought to enhance partnership. Also, instead of trying to overpower client doubts by presenting information or other persuasive strategies, this helper listened to and reflected back the client's ambivalence. First, the helper intuited how the client may potentially feel if parental fighting occurred. That is a highlight of reflective listening. The helper used another reflection to attempt to generate change talk. When the helper used the reflection, "You could see that backfiring and are pretty sure nothing good would come out of it," notice how the client responded by saying that there may actually be some benefits to a family session. That is change talk. Finally, notice that, although a decision was not reached, the helper accepts the client, telling them that they will support them no matter what.

THE FOUR TASKS OF MI

Miller and Rollnick (2012) distinguished four overlapping tasks, including engaging, focusing, evoking, and planning. Clinicians cycle through these tasks, which dynamically recur throughout helping relationships. Engaging refers to building a positive working alliance with clients (i.e., rapport, working alliance). Miller and Rollnick (2012) consider initial engagement as the bedrock for all that follows during MI. However, in the context of family work, engagement may repeat if new family members are introduced during the course the relationship with the helper. Focusing refers to clearly defining the help that is wanted. It has to do with the "what" of change. Evoking refers to evoking change talk around the family goal. Thus, one can think of this as conversing about the "why" of change. This has always been central to MI, given that embedded in the definition of MI is the explicit mention of resolving client ambivalence. In situations where ambivalence about change is not a quintessential feature of the client's presentation, evoking is less important. Finally, planning involves the "how" of change. As noted above, when clients talk about actions they will pursue en route to change, it is a special form of change talk (i.e., commitment, activation, taking steps) thought to reflect a high level of motivation.

Yet, these tasks are not linear, and family work is sometimes messy. For example, you may develop a congenial relationship with a family (i.e., engagement), collaboratively clarify what a family wants (i.e., focusing on improving communication), beautifully elicit why it is important to change within the family's broader goals (i.e., evoking), and develop strategies they are willing to try (i.e. planning). However, as is sometimes the case, one family member may renege on the goal and not pursue communication strategies initially agreed upon. Other members may be hurt and want you to confront the family member to get them to change. This may trigger the helper to circle back to engaging or evoking. Alternatively, a helper may establish a brilliant connection to a family member, only to have a bad day at work and do something inadvertently that fractures rapport. The helper may need to revisit engagement. Thus, the tasks overlap and may need revisiting.

In summary, the four tasks represent a heuristic for how MI proceeds during the course of any helping relationship. They overlap and are often nonlinear. Finally, it is important to note that MI can be used during all four tasks. Because the four tasks mimic common helping phases found in family work, subsequent chapters delve into them in greater detail (see Chapters 9 and 10).

SUMMARY

MI addresses client ambivalence throughout the course of helping relationships. Yet, paradoxically, helpers should not view it as a way to "get their clients" to do what they want them to do, or they risk offering only faux autonomy respect. High-quality MI involves the masterful use of micro-counseling skills, where they seamlessly address all aspects of the method's overarching spirit (i.e., partnership, acceptance, compassion, empowerment) discussed in the next chapter. Increasingly complex reflective listening can address multiple MI spirit dimensions simultaneously. Thus, every interaction represents an opportunity to show deep respect for our client's inner worth and current dilemma while gently nudging toward change. Such nudging occurs by evoking client change language in the broader context of a warm, empathic relationship.

MI requires genuine respect of clients' autonomy.

CHAPTER 3

The Spirit of Motivational Interviewing

Rules are often an excuse to ignore compassion.
—Frank Herbert

There is little question that family-centered care works. However, its effectiveness will largely hinge on how well the provider implements it. In fact, science shows us that, when we directly compare the outcomes of two treatments that are both reputable and well supervised, they usually produce equivalent results (Wampold & Imel, 2015). Although family-centered care has a strong rationale and is grounded in evidence, *how* it is delivered matters a great deal.

Mastering the techniques associated with family-centered care forms only part of the puzzle. Restructuring family communications, educating members about particular health problems, or increasing parental monitoring of their teenage children's whereabouts are all valuable pieces. These tasks could be done with a heavy or light hand. Creating warm environments matters a great deal.

One axiom taught in all training programs is that helpers must develop rapport with their clients. But what exactly does that mean? What does it look like to develop a therapeutic alliance or be empathic? Through many years of experience training MSW students and supervising practitioners, I've encountered a lot of folk wisdom about the meaning of these terms. For example, some helpers think you can develop a solid helper/client relationship through self-disclosure. Others feel compelled to display their knowledge of a client's worldview in terms of their music or culture. An example of this is a helper working with adolescents who tries to develop rapport by talking extensively about what music the teen enjoys. Maybe I can reach you if I show you that I understand some basic facts about your cultural or generational frame of reference? Sometimes, however, this approach simply does not reduce the social and generational distance between a helper and a suspicious, autonomy-seeking youngster. In family-centered care, there is a lot of emphasis on joining with the family and hearing everyone's perspective. Yet, it is critical to remember that these strategies are all techniques aimed at creating the atmosphere in which we believe change can occur.

If done mechanically, and without attention to client cues, any technique or treatment package can flop. MI provides helpers with a framework for creating an environment in which change can happen no matter what specific therapeutic models you favor. This environment is often referred to as the underlying spirit of MI. The spirit of MI is broader than the specific techniques. It is more like a worldview from which helpers approach clients, which drives all their actions.

With MI, change can happen within any therapeutic model.

The purpose of this chapter is to describe this overarching feel of MI. As noted earlier, key components of MI Spirit include partnership, acceptance, compassion, and empowerment. Brief definitions of each of these components appear in Table 3.1.

ATTENDING TO THE MI SPIRIT

Why is it important to focus on the general spirit with which we deliver MI? Consider text messaging. Conversations happening via text messaging are often prone to misunderstandings, often resulting from a lack of context. Just as texted words could lose their meaning absent some well-placed emojis or a shared history of trust with the sender, so, too, do clinical techniques. Well-intentioned statements made by helpers may simply rouse suspicions of their intentions without the appropriate context. Helpers could say all the right words, but without the right spirit, families may question what they mean or what they are after.

When listening to recorded role-plays submitted by students in my classes, I occasionally hear students that have mastered some of the techniques inherent to MI such as reflective listening or open questioning (see Chapter 4). However, the reflections or open questions they use sometimes miss the mark on fostering a sense of partnership, compassion, acceptance or empowerment. An example would be the open question "What types of

TABLE 3.1. Dimensions of the MI Spirit

Component	Definition	Do this . . .	Not this . . .
Partnership	The helper explicitly seeks and values family input in all phases of the relationship.	• Ask what would be helpful. • Ask permission to give advice. • Respect a client's ideas about how change should occur.	• Rigidly adhere to an agenda. • Tell families what to do. • Give unsolicited advice.
Acceptance	The helper respects the family's inherent worth no matter what the circumstances.	• Present ideas as choices. • Use reflections to show you can walk in their shoes.	• Limit your family's choices • Listen haphazardly. • Confront clients.
Compassion	The helper holds the family's interests above all else.	• Understand your motives. • Keep them in check.	• Think that MI can get clients to do what you want them to do.
Empowerment	The helper builds upon family strengths to foster self-efficacy and self-determination.	• Highlight client strengths. • Guide toward informed decisions about behavior change. • Foster opportunities to master skills.	• Supply all the ideas. • Take credit for the family's successes.

things does your family enjoy doing together?" In and of itself, this could be a great question. In addition, when viewed as a technical skill, the ability to ask an open question is part of MI proficiency. However, sometimes students use this type of open question for the sole purpose of rapidly setting up prescriptive advice. For example, students often explore with wonderful open questions, only to prematurely make suggestions that rupture alliances with family members. Consider the following brief exchange:

HELPER: Tell me about your day-to-day family life.

PARENT: Well, we seem to pass in the halls a lot. We're so busy racing around and super-stressed by a full schedule.

HELPER: Have you thought about eating more meals together as a family?

In and of itself, the helper's proposition is not horrible. Yet, there are more collaborative ways of discovering solutions, and what happens if the family already tried having family meals together and failed in using that approach? Clients may wonder if the helper will listen to them or help them find solutions they haven't yet pondered. This is exactly why we differentiate between MI listening skills and its underlying spirit. In the example above, we have a technique, an open question, without partnership, a dimension of the MI Spirit I will soon discuss further.

Another example of potentially implementing a treatment without creating a warm environment comes from a curious scientific finding. Specifically, when MI was facilitated by a therapy manual, a guide that standardizes procedures for replicability in science, it produced poorer clinical outcomes (Hettema et al., 2005). This may have been because therapy manuals focus on standardizing an intervention. Like the foul lines on a baseball field, they tell helpers what activities are in and out of bounds, and sometimes the order in which they need to do these activities. In doing so, therapy manuals may inadvertently cause helpers to become overly focused on techniques and more rigid in terms of using clinical judgment when reading queues from family members. In other words, helpers may check off planned activities but deliver them in a rigid or ineffective way. In summary, there may be something about attending to the broader context of the intervention rather than just what techniques are used.

In the pages that follow, I begin by discussing a major antithesis to the MI Spirit, proceeding from an expert stance. Then, I further elaborate on the MI Spirit dimensions of partnership, acceptance, compassion, and empowerment.

THE EXPERT TRAP IN FAMILY WORK

Helping professionals dedicate years of formal training to learning their crafts and, in doing so, absorb mountains of information about the causes and treatments for human suffering. Knowledge of signs and symptoms of distress, derived from empirical research, is supposed to inform our ability to help others. We assume that, once a problem is correctly diagnosed, the matter of fixing it seems self-evident.

To illustrate this point further, Carl Rogers (1961) recounted a story of his personal transformation from working within this expertise-based model toward the client-centered one he famously developed. After unsuccessful efforts to convince a mother of her role in her son's externalizing behavior, an explanation she simply could not accept, Rogers indicated to her that he could do no more for her son. He concluded, based on his sense that he knew what was best, that she simply could not gain insight that her early maternal rejection influenced his behavior, and thus treatment could not proceed. Upon termination, she then asked if Rogers would see her as a client. At that time, he worked primarily with children in a guidance clinic. Upon agreeing to see her, she started extensively self-disclosing about her troubled marriage and personal fears. Over the course of her treatment, the client reported that her son's behavior improved significantly. Rogers learned that shifting from getting this mother to accept his wisdom toward listening to her troubles made all the difference for this family. Similarly, when we helpers force a systemic view of problems to our clients in family-centered care, we may inadvertently create impasses.

Well-intentioned helpers often fall into this very trap that Rogers described 60 years ago. In MI, we refer to this as the **expert trap**, the conviction that we can advise and prescribe our way out of problems if only our clients would let us. We tell ourselves that truth about clinical problems, once it is known, should be rationally and systematically applied. However, when dealing with complex interactions between people, truth is often in the eye of the beholder.

Taking an expert stance with families may tell us more about our personal hidden biases than about families' capacities to change. Specifically, an underlying assumption supporting the expert trap is that people are inherently unable to change without being told what to do. It is deficit-based thinking.

Humanistic approaches, however, such as MI and client-centered therapy, assume that families have resources and strengths to solve their own problems. There is a much more hopeful view of families as self-correcting systems that may only need a nudge from a trusted guide. Thus, helping becomes less about setting people straight or imparting wisdom, and more about harnessing strengths and empowering families. Helpers can integrate research when guiding families toward change if they refrain from weaponizing research or practice experience. In fact, several adaptations of MI integrate normative statistical data from psychological testing and the highly humanistic counseling style encouraged here that privileges families' lived experiences.

The Expert Trap and Family Systems Perspectives

In family-centered care, helpers advocate for a systems perspective. That is, helpers conceptualize problems as stemming from family interactions and want their clients to think about the family system rather than pathology living in one member. As you recall, we often call that singled-out person the identified client. However, what if helpers communicate the systems perspective too forcibly to the family members? It may backfire. That is, if the helper argues for family members to see the problem as a systems problem, and the family members insist that the problem is an individual and not systemic one, impasses arise.

Some impasses like this can simply be avoided if the helper is willing to let go of their need to get clients to accept certain perspectives. The **fixing reflex** occurs when helpers attempt to correct, educate, or instill knowledge in clients. It is a helper's natural reaction to experiencing client disagreement on how to proceed. For example, it is normal to want to rely on one's training and experience, which often guides our focus to problems that need to be remedied. Yet, when said in a way that undermines autonomy or stymies collaboration, these helper attempts may fail.

One example of pushing a diagnosis or perspective comes from family-centered substance use treatment. Some models communicate the family systems view by telling families that addiction is a "family disease." The mistake we make too often, though, is presenting this framing to the family with too much conviction and too early. Consider how this approach would be met by a family that disagrees with this perspective, and maintains that the identified patient, or person with a substance use problem, is mainly responsible for their woes. If we prescribe a model too fast without fostering partnership, we may risk disengagement from treatment.

The alternative to a top-down approach involving a helper's fixing reflex is taking a collaborative stance to build partnership. It blends helper expertise on solving problems with families' input. One way of thinking about this is that helpers and families must meet in the middle on ways to communicate about problems.

Myth Acceptance

To work with clients effectively, we need an agreed-upon way of talking about what the problem is that brought them to therapy, how it came to be, and how it will be resolved. Wampold and Imel (2015) suggest that we need to co-create a shared language system between the client and helper around which they can explain the etiology of problems, rally hope, and describe progress. They refer to this arrival at a shared language system as **myth acceptance**. MI, if done true to spirit, would involve family-centered care workers co-creating a new myth with every new family, rather than imposing a boilerplate myth upon families. In Chapter 4, I will review some of the communication skills that can help with fostering partnership and coming to shared understandings of problems.

Parallels with Parenting

Contemporary thinking on parenting contains some parallels regarding this discussion on the tension between expertise and collaboration. Specifically, authoritative parenting refers to a parenting style where strong balance exists between demonstrating affection and enforcing rules and expectations. Four parenting styles originally articulated by Diana Baumrind (2005) include authoritative, authoritarian, permissive, and neglectful. Whereas authoritative parenting balances warmth with limit setting, authoritarian parents exhibit low warmth and are highly punitive. Permissive parents are warm but do not set or enforce limits. Finally, neglectful parents are low on displaying warmth as well as overt attempts to shape their children's behaviors. Baumrind's parenting model has been extensively studied with parents of adolescents, and the benefits of authoritative parenting are well established (Steinberg, 2001).

In my prior research, I considered whether changes in authoritative parenting influenced substance use among adolescents in treatment (Smith & Hall, 2008). I was also interested in whether more exposure to family therapy would lead to better reductions in adolescent substance use. I was crushed when my hypothesis didn't work, but it was a life-changing experience for me as a clinical scientist because it forced me to think more deeply about my assumptions of how people change and come to the perspective that there are multiple pathways to good outcomes.

Of course, there are many differences between parenting and being a helping professional. Professional boundaries come to mind. On the other hand, it does not seem so far-fetched to compare children's reactions to an expert but judgmental helper to those of an overly controlling parent who does not display much affection. If professional expertise is doled out in the absence of a trusting, warm relationship, it may fail. Just as parents often describe "picking their battles" with their children, helpers should consider when it is critical to express expertise.

Doling out expertise in the absence of a trusting, warm relationship is wasted effort.

As well, there may be times when helping professionals may lean too much toward warmth and acceptance of their clients—acting similarly to permissive parents. This posture may leave their clients wondering when they will actually do any therapeutic work. In fact, studies exist showing that some professional helpers err in this direction and are perceived by their clients as overly chatty and nonprofessional (Audet & Everall, 2010). In short, MI Spirit and its therapeutic techniques need to be balanced for optimal effects.

EXPERTISE AND AMBIVALENCE ABOUT CHANGE

What is it about sharing expertise with clients that sometimes creates impasses? Who would knowingly reject a rational and well-researched plan for ameliorating a problem? Let us start off by asking ourselves if it is really that unusual for families to second guess our expertise in providing systemic, family-centered care. Clients may be thinking that therapy may work for others, but what about their family? Even as experts, we must acknowledge that research on empirically supported treatments reports the average effects. Not all families benefit, even if the averaged net benefits are positive. A certain degree of humility seems in order. As professionals, we have vast knowledge of what generally helps families thrive, but not necessarily whether it will work for the particular family in front of us.

A critical part of avoiding the communication of smug expertise is assessing what families have already tried. Consider the perspective of a family that has been disappointed by previous attempts of systemic therapy, only to be told to try it again. Many professionals will merely explain to the family that their past treatment was a failure because they didn't truly engage with the therapy. This is essentially communicating that the treatment is not wrong, the family is.

Overreliance on expertise may trigger or possibly strengthen family members' ambivalence about whether or how change should occur. As we discussed in the Chapter 1, hesitation about change occurs naturally. Some apprehension among family members about working with helpers should be expected. Families may be wondering if working with a helper is worth the effort, such as the emotional risks involved with talking candidly about painful family interactions. They may fear the potential ramifications of seeing a helper whom they were mandated to see, wondering if the helper is merely an appendage of some carceral system. Families can be ambivalent about whether change should occur, and also how change should occur. Overshooting from an expert stance may trigger or even intensify this ambivalence and contribute to families deciding to leave care before any benefits accrue.

PARTNERSHIP

The antidote to taking an expert stance is striving in all communications to build a partnership with family members, where their expertise is actively sought and valued. Instead of operating from the perspective that one's expertise will drive the process, helpers who successfully use MI foster deep partnerships with families. They use their expertise only when needed, and largely as a supplement to the strengths and resources brought in by the families they see. To draw once more on the work of Carl Rogers (1961), building a partnership involves a shift in thinking from "how I can treat this family" toward "how I can be of assistance to them." In other words, it is a shift from getting the family to accept your view of the problem toward coming to a mutual understanding of it.

MI is done with, and not *to*, families. Families that sense treatments are being done to them may choose to leave prematurely or resent the helper's efforts as manipulative. Families should never feel like we are secretly trying to manipulate them to do things about which they are currently ambivalent. MI does not trick resistant people into change (Miller & Rollnick, 2009). Instead, its practitioners develop partnerships and actively call upon family expertise in discussions about change.

Another descriptor that is often used to refer to partnership is power sharing, which involves things like deferring to the family's preference for the agenda of each session, setting aside your plans if something more urgent or important to the family arises, and being not too wedded to activities that you consider critical if they collide with families' wishes. I particularly like the practice of some family-based interventions that open each session asking what the client wants to discuss but where helpers have a plan if the client voices no priorities. This tactic avoids the uncomfortable predicament of providing too little structure in the name of emphasizing partnership.

Examples of overt efforts to exert power, which are contraindicated in MI, include appealing to fear or shame to convince family members to act, confronting a family's ideas as unreasonable, or building up your authority as an expert when persuading a family to do something. Imagine a therapist saying, "You know, I've been doing this a long time, so I can tell you that the path your family is on is dangerous. If you all want to be estranged from each other, just keep on doing what you're doing." Such a statement is confrontational and fundamentally different from what we mean by evocation and partnership.

Partnership is not merely the absence of overt and highly patronizing techniques that undermine family input. It is actively looking for opportunities to gather the wisdom of the family. Some common strategies include asking the family what they want to prioritize, asking the family how they want to go about meeting goals before giving our suggestions, and affirming the family's ideas. Another strategy is directly telling families, nonpossessively, that they can always choose whether or not they will change or follow any suggestions you may give.

> **Partnership is actively looking for opportunities to gather the wisdom of the family.**

One benefit of working on developing partnerships is that they tend to be more generative and efficient than models where advice is given from the expert stance. That is, when helpers give unsolicited advice that family members don't think is feasible or attractive (e.g., increase family meals), time may be spent discussing why that is not a good solution. It incurs an opportunity cost where, at minimum, a few moments of time have been wasted and, at worst, it results in a small rupture in the therapeutic alliance. Furthermore, if families generate their own solutions, they can be credited to the family's efforts or resourcefulness. That is, helpers can affirm their efforts and increase their sense of self-efficacy in solving their problems.

ACCEPTANCE

Myriad definitions of acceptance exist. Here, we are referring to helpers accepting families, not families accepting expert advice, accepting reality as it is, or accepting the present moment as practiced in mindfulness-based approaches. Acceptance involves treating all families as people with inherent worth, whether helpers agree or disagree with their values, decisions, or actions—taking families as they are, not how the helper would like them to be. It means taking a nonjudgmental stance in all communications with families.

The importance of accepting families as they are cannot be overstated. Without feeling accepted by their helpers, it is hard to see how personal growth or change can occur. A fundamental stance of acceptance toward the client provides the secure attachment required to facilitate the hard work that therapy entails. It frees families to speak candidly and take risks in the presence of a third party.

Many challenges exist for helpers to achieve such a stance. If you've had training in a marriage and family therapy program or another helping profession, you've likely been exposed to client activities where you examined your personal beliefs. Examples of personal beliefs that may hinder accepting families include our values about parenting, whether a family should keep an elder at home, or the morality of open relationships. Accepting others with values different from our own is a challenge, but it is essential to practicing within the spirit of MI.

Communicating acceptance requires maintaining composure. Helpers who live in the moment, who can demonstrate a high level of acceptance, have learned how to filter out any negative personal reactions that arise. Few helpers want to be perceived as judgmental or nonaccepting. They may, however, get rattled and unintentionally say something that is heard as judgmental, or display a facial expression that communicates disapproval of the family. Or, in light of challenges in a session, they could simply spend less session time highlighting family strengths or making statements that express positive regard (that is, affirmations, which we will discuss in Chapter 4). Fortunately, with practice, every interaction can desensitize us to such challenging stimuli.

Sometimes clients will tell helpers that an accepting atmosphere exists in their sessions together. Families may verbalize "feeling heard," "listened to," "not judged," "respected," "surprised by focusing on strengths instead of problems," or "valued" to name a few.

COMPASSION

The word "compassion" derives from the Latin roots *com* and *pati*, which when combined, translate roughly to "with suffering." Broadly speaking then, compassion is defined here as a nonpossessive effort to help alleviate someone else's suffering: to be with their suffering, to acknowledge it and offer understanding and help, to have their pain and suffering take center stage.

Miller and Rollnick (2012) discussed an urgent need to ground MI in compassion. Specifically, over the course of many years of training, they became upset with some applications of MI that were being used to attempt to get people to do things that people in the helping profession have no business persuading clients to do. Thus, MI explicitly focuses on what the clients perceive as their best outcomes, rather than what clinicians see.

MI focuses on what the *clients* perceive as their best outcomes.

Cultivating Compassion

Training that focuses on environmental influences on family behavior may help cultivate compassion for families. One of the things I've always valued about social work training is that it focuses on environmental factors. Per accreditation standards, marital and family therapy programs do as well (Commission on Accreditation for Marriage and Family Therapy Education, 2021). I wonder if helpers would express more compassion if they dwelled on the impacts of poverty, joblessness, and discrimination on family members' behaviors.

In a similar manner, developing knowledge about internal biological states or developmental stages may also influence helpers to stay grounded in compassion. Messaging about certain mental health disorders, including addictions, often focuses on the biological nature as part of a deliberate strategy to reduce public stigma. Does this framing also facilitate compassion among helpers? Similarly, remembering that adolescents and younger children lack certain experiences, or require further prefrontal cortex maturation, may prove beneficial in centering helpers on having compassion. When we recognize that certain things are out of the control of, and stressful to, families, it seems that helpers can foster compassion a little easier.

Another promising way to develop compassion involves structured meditations focusing on loving kindness (Bibeau et al., 2016). Such meditations involve visualizing a person and wishing them well during mindfulness practice and increase empathy and prosocial behaviors (Luberto et al., 2018). To my knowledge, there are no studies yet showing that clinicians who practice loving-kindness meditations achieve higher ratings for compassion during their MI practice. Yet, helpers who are interested in increasing their compassion for families may consider experimenting with meditations focusing on loving kindness. (See the Appendix for mindfulness-based loving-kindness resources.)

Threats to Compassion

Focusing on the personal responsibility of family members, while driven from a moral perspective, may be a threat to fostering and communicating compassion. For example, a teenage child may have had multiple instances of using marijuana while on probation, forbidden under its terms. Yet, upon further exploration, a helper may find that the youth lives in a small roach-infested apartment with his auntie and mother, with the former recovering from cancer. From a pure legal and moralistic perspective, the child did something wrong. Yet, a compassionate approach would involve understanding the painful context, being with that pain, and helping the child and family work through it. Taking a moral or personal responsibility view without further exploration of the family's underlying pain could result in treatment devoid of compassion.

I also wonder if helpers can become less compassionate through certain feedback loops. For example, from psychological research, we know that attribution errors increase depression (Abramson et al., 1989). That is, individuals who attribute failure to personal traits versus external factors become more depressed (e.g., "I'm a loser" vs. "I didn't do well because I got a bad night's sleep"). Similarly, I wonder if helpers attribute therapeutic failure to families, rather than their own personal behaviors. Families would then serve as an external versus intrinsic attribution or, put more simply—they would be blamed for poor treatment outcomes (i.e., "It's the family, not my approach"). Alternatively, when a helper makes an internal attribution, it would involve taking responsibility for their practices that may have contributed to the therapeutic outcome (i.e., "I need to change my approach"). Making external attributions protects helpers psychologically, shielding them from any uncomfortable feelings associated with needing to increase their compassion for families.

Within the MI literature, there are several tools for monitoring one's own practice behaviors to shift the focus on what we can control (see Appendix for detailed descriptions). Perhaps only after achieving initial mastery and then completing ongoing monitoring of helping behaviors should helpers consider making external attributions for lack of family engagement of negative outcomes. When focused on what helpers can control to engage with and help families, practice evaluation is, in fact, an exercise in maintaining compassion.

In whatever manner helpers cultivate and maintain compassion for clients, it is central to MI. The desire to be of help and not steer toward one's personal agenda is of paramount importance.

EMPOWERMENT

Ultimately, we do not want families to rely on our services indefinitely. Instead, most clinical models seek to enhance their families' capacity for self-management, often called empowerment. Zimmerman (2000) defined an empowered person as one who harbors a sense of personal control, remains aware of their environment, and behaves in a way that enhances their sense of control. At an interpersonal level, couples could be empowered to communicate better or master their personal fight-or-flight responses during arguments (Fishbane, 2011), skills they can use long after their relationship with the helper ends. Empowerment may look slightly different in diverse family-centered care contexts.

Empowerment is often associated with efforts to help oppressed, marginalized, and stigmatized families. Those who have been dealt a rough hand feel powerless and are told that their failures are their fault. Empowerment theorists have thus focused on marginalized gender identities and racial and ethnic minorities from low-income communities.

MI is uplifting and never meant to further oppress or marginalize families. Through careful listening to families' stories, reflection of client statements, and deliberate attempts to create equal partnerships, MI nudges toward empowering families. Students in my classes often remark that they like how reflective listening inherent to MI "makes clients think" or "puts the ball in their court." Students recognize MI as a concrete clinical strategy for empowering clients.

Families experiencing multiple failures are especially in need of empowerment. Among them, there is a natural tendency to give up when they perceive that nothing they do will make a difference. Consider the long road ahead of a mother who has fought a serious opioid addiction and already lost multiple children to the child protection system and just gave birth to another substance-exposed baby. When failure occurs despite the families' perceptions of putting their best efforts forward, it can lead to what psychologists refer to as learned helplessness (Seligman, 1972). Families that have experienced learned helplessness may present with a "Why bother?" attitude. They may express the most sincere desire to change, yet at their core, not believe that they are able to effect change (see the box below).

Working Hard with Families Is Empowering

One concern I have with the term "empowerment" is that helpers may weaponize this concept to shift responsibility onto clients in a punitive manner. It strikes me as strange that even a concept as benign as "empowerment" may be misused in practice. It appears commonplace to hear helpers say that they "will not work harder than their clients." I wonder if this phenomenon is driven by a misunderstanding of the concept of empowerment. That is, helpers seem to use this statement when they are shifting accountability away from themselves and toward the family for therapy outcomes. When helpers work hard with families, it is both compassionate and empowering. This brings us to our next point, that there is overlap among the MI Spirit dimensions.

OVERLAP AMONG MI SPIRIT DIMENSIONS

Partnership, acceptance, compassion, and empowerment are not mutually exclusive categories. For example, in describing empowerment in clinical practice, Zimmerman (2000) specifically linked empowerment to collaboration with partners, rather than experts treating clients. Thus, there can possibly be no empowerment without partnership. Structural family therapists have also noted that respect for autonomy and partnership are critical aspects of empowerment. Finally, when families generate solutions to their own problems in partnership with their helper, they are being empowered. Helpers can later affirm that their efforts and ingenuity led to change, further reinforcing a sense of personal mastery and control.

SUMMARY

MI seeks to create fertile soil where change can take root. Creating that soil requires that we practice partnership, acceptance, compassion, and empowerment, which are components of the spirit of MI. In many ways, they intertwine with the techniques of MI, to which we will now turn our attention.

CHAPTER 4

ROARS Skills

> When people talk, listen completely.
> Most people never listen.
> —Ernest Hemingway

MI is talk therapy. Thus, we achieve the spirit of MI and work to resolve ambivalence about change through specific things we say to families. Many clinicians know the nuts and bolts of MI as *active listening, reflective listening,* or *micro-counseling* skills. These skills include open questions, affirmations, reflections, and summaries. OARS is the often-used acronym used to describe these skills collectively within the MI community. However, as MI increasingly emphasizes reflections, and the quality of reflections is an indicator of MI mastery, I suggest that we consider elevating the "R." Thus, at the risk of committing acronym heresy, I refer to these skills in this book collectively as the ROARS skills, including reflections, open questions, affirmations, and reflective summaries.

The terminology used to describe these skills differs across counseling texts among the various helping professions. Therefore, in this chapter, I attempt to link various terms to those used in the family-centered care and general counseling literatures.

ARE YOU ALREADY DOING MI?

Helpers sometimes have fundamental misunderstandings of what the ROARS skills are or have not sufficiently developed them to use in a manner consistent with MI. Many treatment providers say they are already doing MI. However, my personal observations of helpers I've trained has left me questioning that. For example, I once encountered a trainee who swore they were using reflective listening yet did not use a single reflection when asked to role-play. Instead, they demonstrated a skill used sparingly in MI, closed questioning. Furthermore, we know that self-reported skill level in MI does not match up with neutral observers' ratings (Beckman et al., 2022). So, it is important to clearly define the ROARS and talk about what differentiates use of ROARS in MI versus the use of ROARS in other helping models.

Although many helpers already use ROARS, the use of these skills varies on two critical fronts: skillfulness and strategic purpose. Helpers using MI demonstrate a high level of skillfulness in using ROARS and also use them for very specific purposes. Specifically, we use ROARS to both build an atmosphere in which change can occur and evoke change talk. We discussed the former at length in Chapter 3 and will discuss the latter at length in Chapter 5.

Skillful Use of ROARS

Some types of ROARS are much simpler to master than others. Some general considerations when thinking about the skillfulness with which someone is using ROARS include clarity, awareness of cultural and developmental nuances about communications, and voice tone.

New helpers often use jargon-laden phrases that may be less impactful than simpler, clearer language. For example, consider the two reflections said in response to a client talking about difficulties in changing their eating when those around them incessantly snack on unhealthy foods. Both reflections attempt to communicate the same thing:

> *Example 1 (jargon):* "It sounds like your social network has some toxic elements to it, and you're thinking about what it will take to sustain changes in your behavior. You cannot have that working against you."
>
> *Example 2 (parsimonious):* "For change to stick, you know you'll need supportive people around you."

Err toward parsimony when talking to families. That is, try to find the simplest, clearest way to say things so that people can understand you. Kurt Vonnegut, a well-regarded American author, famously wrote an essay where one of his writing tips was to "pity the reader" (Vonnegut, 1985). His point was that clarity and simplicity often win the day and make for more pleasant communication. As helpers, we, too, should think about clear communication.

Another example where parsimony may be achieved is by avoiding unnecessarily long windups. These may work against our message and get lost in translation by the client due to us speaking too long. For example, many helpers have learned that, unless we add stems like "It sounds like . . . ," "It seems like . . . ," "I'm sensing that . . . ," or "I just want to check this out because what I hear you saying is . . . ," we are putting words in client's mouths when reflecting. However, this is often not the case. Clients appear to respond well to simple, crisp reflections without the need for long windups.

Clarity and simplicity win the day.

Heeding cultural and developmental nuances is also critical (Lee, 2025). One of my former MI trainers noted how affirmations should be used sparingly in her culture due to the reserved nature of her countrymen. So, some affirmations or compliments may actually be distressing to individuals from cultures that are a bit more reserved, valuing social distance and casual small talk, rather than affirmations like, "You are doing an amazing job. I appreciate you so much."

Developmental factors also matter. When working with families, we need to attend to whether the wording we're using is accessible by children or older adults. (Specifically, consider developmental factors such as cognitive ability or age-related historical frames of reference.) For example, youth are still learning abstract thinking skills, so using concrete examples can often be beneficial. Consider the following things said to a 13-year-old who enjoys superhero movies and is experiencing extreme sadness:

Example 1 (more abstract): "How does that make you feel?"

Example 2 (more concrete): "You feel like that superhero's daughter right after he died. It's that intense."

Of course, this statement would never work with someone who did not see the referenced film. So, using such statements should be limited to scenarios where you think it will land. Remember, the key point with this concrete statement in the example above was that it could possibly make an abstract feeling (i.e., sadness or depression) more concrete to a young person by using a specific type of event that would make someone sad.

It may help them process through the emotion easier if they are given an example to compare their feeling against versus the more challenging task of describing an abstract sensation from scratch.

Finally, many of us were taught to use a "warm" voice tone. Indeed, voice tone can dramatically impact whether family members perceive certain ROARS skills as threatening. On the other hand, practicing MI is not acting. It is not saying your lines and expecting a result. There is not a "therapy voice" that differs from one's everyday voice. The art of learning ROARS skills involves using skills deliberately but conversationally, as if you were talking to one of your own friends or family members.

These three dimensions of clarity, cultural and developmental awareness, and vocal tone are at the core of skillful MI practice. For example, how can you be empathic without speaking with families in a way that acknowledges cultural and developmental nuances? How can partnership be developed if the helper is perceived as abrupt or confuses the family with lengthy speeches?

Strategic Use of ROARS

Strategic, rather than willy-nilly, use of ROARS moves helpers closer to a mindful and empathic way of being with families. The use of ROARS can be called *strategic* when these micro-counseling skills convey the MI Spirit or are deliberately used to work toward resolving ambivalence. Helpers may be using a ROARS skill, but with no identifiable link to the underlying spirit of MI. In MI, ROARS skills are used deliberately and strategically to build a strong partnership, enhance autonomy, and elicit and reinforce a family's motivation for change. Thus, we can often judge the utility of helpers' ROARS skills in light of the underlying spirit of MI that we discussed in Chapter 3. For example, when we ask questions, we can consider whether they serve well for building a partnership, emphasizing autonomy, expressing acceptance, or displaying compassion. ROARS skills are also used to resolve ambivalence, which we will discuss further in Chapter 5.

ROARS skills are used deliberately and strategically.

One statement made by a helper can map onto multiple components of the MI Spirit. I call these **multipurpose statements**. The difference between good MI and great MI is how efficiently a helper can use such statements and thereby communicate multiple aspects of the MI Spirit through the micro-counseling skills they employ.

ROARS

Reflective Listening (R)

A reflection is a statement that plays off something your client said or something nonverbal that you observed. Statements are not questions, just observations that may contain guesses about what is going on. Consider the following two examples that demonstrate how reflections differ from questions and are always yoked to a client statement:

Example 1: Response with a Question
FAMILY MEMBER: I'm so sick of how they all treat me.
HELPER: Can you give me an example of what they are doing?

Example 2: Reflective Response
FAMILY MEMBER: I'm so sick of how they all treat me.
HELPER: You want them to treat you better, and you're hoping we can do something together about this.

    Furthermore, reflections are generally not questions that seek specific information. Therefore, reflections by definition do not start with the stems "Do you . . . ?," "Can you . . . ?," "Did you . . . ?," "Have you . . . ?," or "Will you . . . ?" Instead, reflections are statements that either paraphrase, rephrase or otherwise react to something your client just said. When done well, reflections offer the highest level of tangible proof of helpers' empathy and compassion.
    Simple reflections only serve one purpose or stay close to the client's verbiage. Many simple reflections, like the statement "You seem frustrated," serve a beneficial purpose in terms of building rapport and communicating empathy. Simple reflections are valuable. Simple reflections can be used to communicate empathy when clients express intense emotion or are severely agitated (e.g., "You're furious"). Sometimes helpers also just need time to think about the client's situation, and simple reflections may be easier to do. However, when simple reflections are overused, they often can leave a conversation in a kind of eddy, not moving forward. To illustrate this, I will use an example of responding with only simple reflections and then an example of using more complex ones. Consider the case where one partner in a romantic relationship has reservations about their loved one going back to school.

Example 1: *Standing Still Because of Repeated Use of Simple Reflections*

FAMILY MEMBER: I think, if she goes back to school, we'll never see each other.

HELPER: You'll never get to talk.

FAMILY MEMBER: Yes, it will really hurt our relationship.

HELPER: The relationship will suffer.

FAMILY MEMBER: yes, it will.

HELPER: This is a difficult time for you.

FAMILY MEMBER: Yeah, it is. I don't know how we let ourselves get here.

HELPER: And you want things to be different.

FAMILY MEMBER: Yeah, I want us to be close again.

Example 2: *Getting Deeper with Complex Reflections*

FAMILY MEMBER: I think, if she goes back to school, we'll never see each other.

HELPER: You don't want to be just roommates.

FAMILY MEMBER: Exactly. We're already not talking much, and this will worsen things.

HELPER: Things are strained. It's not that you don't want them to have a fulfilling career, you just worry about the timing.

FAMILY MEMBER: Maybe if I felt a little closer to them, I'd have an easier time with this.

HELPER: You know you need to let them follow their dreams, and you also don't want to lose what makes you special as a couple in the process.

FAMILY MEMBER: Yeah, of course I love them and want them to be happy. But we're not in a good place. We used to be so close. We talked for hours and hours and then drifted apart when our careers took off.

HELPER: Adjusting to that is hard, and you want to make it through this more demanding time. It's one thing you want to work on.

FAMILY MEMBER: Yes, I think that would be a great starting place.

In the examples above, the first one used a series of four simpler reflections, and this resulted in a shallower conversation. The family member did not expand as much to these simple reflections, in part because they stayed so close to what was already said. However, in the second example, the client responded with more information. This is because the clinician used the reflections to highlight both the underlying emotions of the client, as well as emphasize certain parts of their statements.

Complex reflections add some pizazz. Thus, they are often used for deepening conversations that feel stuck. A therapist may want to emphasize a particular part of what the family member said to take the conversation in a particular direction. Consider the statement above in the second example, "You don't want to be just roommates." Roommates should have less intimacy and more independence than strong romantic couples. So, this was a creative way of taking a guess that they want something more than that—they want intimacy! Note what the client said immediately prior to this. They said, "... we'll never see each other." The helper went on out on a limb here that the underlying feeling was one of how intimacy may suffer by becoming busier. Importantly, it wasn't said by the client. It was evoked through a complex reflection.

Complex reflections deepen conversations.

In addition to deepening conversations, complex reflections are also excellent for resolving some ambivalence (which we will expand on in Chapter 5). For example, complex reflections often expand the dialogue. Consider the difference between "You seem frustrated" and "You're frustrated by being here, and yet you came." Both hit on the frustration, but the second reflection adds emphasis about the client's potential motivation for attending. By merely adding six words, the reflection morphed into a multipurpose statement, both conveying empathy and evoking motivation.

Table 4.1 contrasts examples of questions with examples of reflections, both in response to the same family member behavior shown in the leftmost column. Notice how the reflections are more likely to be multipurpose statements.

Reflective listening serves as a signpost to families that you understand their situation, which is essentially the definition of empathy. Ideally, family members will sense that you are fully there with them, listening with care. Also, reflective listening is efficient. People often think of questions as the most efficient way of extracting information. But often, we can get information organically in the course of a genuine conversation. It is harder to build rapport through a cyclical pattern of asking and receiving answers to questions. When you prioritize reflective listening in your work, families are less likely to sense that you are trying to manipulate them or control their behavior. This is exactly because reflections play off what the family said. Notice in the second example above how practically all the complex reflections included the word "you," referring to the client. Specifically, reflections do not communicate *the helper's* opinion, desires for the client, or agenda. Questions, on the other hand, can often be perceived as communicating an agenda. Thus, reflections are less likely to provoke strong reactions from family members that may create clinical impasses. Finally, reflections hold a special role in resolving ambivalence, which we will further discuss in Chapter 5 and subsequent chapters.

Because of the clinical benefits of reflections, and their role in helpers' being mindfully present, they hold a privileged place in MI. Training standards for MI specify the ideal of achieving a ratio of two reflections per question asked. Furthermore, complex reflections should comprise roughly 50% of all a helper's reflections (Moyers et al., 2016). Thus, when reading longer mock dialogues in the remainder of this book, I encourage you to look at the examples of complex reflections, meditating on what, and how many, purposes they serve.

TABLE 4.1. Contrasting Questions with Reflections

Clinical context	Question(s)	Reflection
You notice the nonverbal behaviors of two members of a couple that indicate anger.	"Tell me about why you two look so angry today."	"Things seem tense today." [Simple reflection] "You two seem angry today, and yet you came. So, perhaps you're a tiny bit hopeful that you're going to get through this." [Complex reflection, evocation, and empathy]
Client says including his parents in family session would devolve into shouting match.	"What are you worried about happening?"	"Bringing your parents in would be stressful." [Simple reflection] "You could really see that backfiring and are pretty darn sure nothing good would come out of it." [Complex reflection)]
Client says family involvement could potentially help.	"What kinds of things would you like to get off your chest?" "How would you feel if you got those things off your chest?"	"So, it may be worth risking if you could get me in your corner for some things. And it would help you to get some things off your chest." [Complex reflection]

Open Questions (O)

Open questions, as the label suggests, are those that are most likely to broaden the conversation, adding exploratory depth. They are contrasted with closed questions, which usually generate short replies or seek specific, often factual, information.

A principal concern in using questions, or any skill really, is where it takes the conversation. For example, in MI we specifically seek to avoid a pattern where a clinician asks a question, receives a short reply from a family member, and then asks another question. Such a pattern may take on the feel of an interrogation and may start to slip away from the collaborative venture that is MI.

To families that are especially leery about the helping process, it may feel as if each question asked represents a value or assumption about change held by the helper. A family could interpret a series of questions as the helper's trying to get out all the relevant facts, so they can prescribe a predetermined solution in an expert fashion. If a family identifies this happening, they may react negatively, and the conversation may devolve into the **question–answer trap**, whereby the family members respond with nothing but short answers. This may be in direct response to the information being sought, or, worse, as a mechanism to preserve their privacy or dignity. Consider the following short example:

HELPER: When did your family's troubles start?
FAMILY MEMBER: It's been happening for some time.
HELPER: Okay. And is it better or worse when it is winter?
FAMILY MEMBER: Neither really.
HELPER: And is it worse or better when you all eat together as a family?
FAMILY MEMBER: Neither.
HELPER: And have you tried to work on your communication skills?
FAMILY MEMBER: Not really . . . no.

Notice how the conversation appears to be contracting rather than expanding. It is stuck on the task of collection of information. As mentioned earlier, the family can sometimes see right through where a clinician is going if they ask specific questions such as, "Is it better or worse in the winter?" This question implies that a problem may be seasonal, and savvy families may wonder if the clinician is assessing for affective disorders that occur in the winter in some regions. If this misses the mark, however, or a family member does not like the idea of having seasonal depression, it may provoke a short reply. This is not necessarily resistance. Instead, it seems like a natural response for a family member who senses that time is being wasted on dead-end streets. In short, some questions may fail if they trigger families to consider whether a helper has an underlying agenda. In that situation, they may react negatively with short replies, reinforcing a cyclical impasse.

Alternatively, open questions are expansive and generative. Let's consider the following different approach:

HELPER: Why did your family come in today?

FAMILY MEMBER: Well, we are really struggling. I called because we just can't seem to stop fighting. We are under a lot of stress, all feeling cooped up under the same room since the pandemic started. We all feel lonely and distant, even though we are together all the time.

HELPER: It sounds like you want to improve your communication and sense of togetherness. Tell me more about what's going on.

As you can see, a shift in the structure of a question can make a big difference. A few things bear mentioning about this example. First, students are sometimes trained not to ask questions starting with the word "why." This adage only refers to questions that challenge clients prematurely, or in a threatening manner. An example would be using the question "Why do you think that?" Indeed, such direct challenges to someone's internal expertise are often viewed as confrontational and are to be avoided in MI. However, there is no general rule that you avoid "why?" questions in MI as long as the questions don't clash with the MI Spirit. In the example directly above, the main intent of the first question is to explore what is happening with the family. Notice, too, that unlike the earlier example that asked for when a problem started, a specific fact, the family member could have gone in any number of directions in response to the opening question in this example. There is no right answer to open questions. Finally, notice that the client talked more than the helper in this short example.

Regarding the principle that questions can either map onto the MI Spirit or not, I would like to provide a few examples of commonly used open questions. Examples include "Tell me your thoughts on that" (partnership), "So, what do you think you'll do?" (autonomy), and "What would be most helpful to you today?" (partnership). Such questions can be used intentionally to foster the spirit of MI.

As noted earlier, closed questions, by contrast, are those that usually generate short replies or specific information. Examples include "Have you thought about telling your mom how much that hurts you?" and "Have I got that right?" There are two notable comments about these questions. I think there is potential for the first question to be heard as a suggestion by a client. If ambivalence exists, it may provoke a "yeah but" reaction from the client, which we generally try to avoid in MI. Remember, we call that sustain talk. Regarding the second question, many helpers have been trained to check in with clients for accuracy (e.g., "Is that right?") and are subsequently afraid of using reflections without checking on their accuracy with such a follow-up question. It is generally accepted in the MI community that these types of "checking questions" are unnecessary. Although well intentioned, checking if your reflection was accurate by following it with a question may inadvertently choke off conversation. For example, your client may not provide an expansive reply and simply respond by saying, "Yes." Or it may just interrupt the rhythm of the conversation and cause you to have to regroup. The beauty of reflections is that, if done well, they encourage the client to continue deepening the conversation and foster a nice conversational rhythm.

Asking whether your reflection was accurate can choke off conversation.

Affirmations (A)

Affirmations are positive comments about a family or family member. They frequently note some strength or positive aspect of the family's behavior that is commendable. Examples include "You've been working hard on this," "You're a bright person and don't need people breathing down your neck to make good decisions," and "You're pretty resourceful. It takes a lot to survive what you've been through." They are used to create a positive atmosphere, to bond with clients, and to highlight and reinforce successes.

Generally speaking, affirmations are most powerful when they are specific, can be genuinely delivered, and are not overused. For example, simply saying "great job" to a family member may be a certain form of cheerleading, but it lacks depth or specificity. It is a missed opportunity to highlight family member's specific successes. Thus, short statements such as "great job" or "impressive" may contribute to a positive environment but may also be less valued by family members. Helpers should also always use affirmations that they can say genuinely. Some affirmations make helpers very uncomfortable or do not come naturally at first. In the box below,

I elaborate a personal example of this from my work with families. Finally, repetitive use of identical affirmations may also lead family members to devalue them or to see them as disingenuous. Varying the content of affirmations can be more impactful, sending a clear message to families that you value their internal strengths and resources.

Another risk regarding affirmations is whether using an affirmation communicates a form of conditional acceptance of the client. As MI is a model that emphasizes choice and partnership, some consideration must be given to whether affirmations communicate the helper's agenda too forcefully.

"Your Kid Is Lucky to Have You."

When directing an adolescent substance use treatment center, I met with parents and their teenage children to collaboratively review initial assessment findings. One stock affirmation for parents, when meeting with them privately, was "Your kid probably isn't thanking you much right now, so let me tell you that your kid is lucky to have you." Although I frequently used a variation of this statement with parents, I think my delivery, more often than not, was genuine. I personally believed it to be true. Parents seemed to respond well to it. At times, I could see a shift in their nonverbal behaviors, or it would result in them more freely discussing their child's problems. At the time, being younger than most parents of adolescents, I felt nervous about working with clients with more life experience than me. For me, it felt like something I could do to put parents at ease. I wanted to send a clear message early in sessions that I was not there to blame them for their child's problems. Plus, I liked it better than attempting to reduce the social distance between me and older individuals in ways that may have risked sounding apologetic about my lack of life experience. And seemingly, it worked more often than not. Other helpers felt that they would be too uncomfortable saying something like that to their clients. I am not sure if they thought it was too hokey, if they didn't believe it to be true of some parents, or if there were other reasons for their discomfort. I'm glad they didn't attempt it if they didn't think it would work for them. Better a sincere affirmation delivered with personal conviction than a scripted, disingenuous one.

THOUGHT QUESTIONS: (1) What affirmations, if any, do you typically avoid? Why?
(2) Sometimes people say they feel like they are acting lines in a play when they use affirmations. What has your experience been with that?

Reflective Summaries (R)

Reflective summaries are thought of as a series of reflections that recapitulate what the family members have said. So, you can think of them as longer reflections that try to tie together themes, close a session, turn the attention to a new topic, or encapsulate a family's entire discussion of their motivations for change. That is, while a reflection may respond to only one client statement, a reflective summary plays off multiple client statements.

Reflective summaries can be used for different purposes. I define **brief refocusing summaries** as those that simply communicate listening and redirect the conversation to new areas. They are typically used when helpers are sifting through a lot of client content and trying to remain focused or when they determine it's best to go somewhere new. **End-of-session summaries** wrap up entire sessions in an organized fashion and refresh everyone's memory of what has been achieved and what issues may lie on the horizon. These may be especially useful for your own memory as a helper. Saying out loud what happened in a session at the end of a session may have the benefit of keeping you organized. Finally, summaries can compassionately nudge a client in the direction of change by reflecting on all the statements a family's made about wanting to change. That is, any statement family members make in the direction of change is referred to as *change talk*. So, these are referred to as **change talk summaries**. We will further elaborate on change talk in Chapter 5.

Reflective summaries can be simple or complex. If helpers do not add any color commentary or emphasis in their summaries, they may trigger comments from clients like "Yes, that's what I just said." That indicates the use of primarily simple reflections in the summary. However, summaries may contain complex reflections used strategically to deepen conversations and touch on elements of the underlying spirit of MI.

Table 4.2 shows the difference between **brief refocusing** (used midsession), **end-of-session**, and **change talk summaries**, as well as a summary that simply echoes the content very closely. When reading these different summaries, try to imagine that the helper using these summaries heard the same exact things from the client leading up to these summary statements.

SUMMARY

MI does not merely entail the use of "good counseling skills," such as the ROARS we have defined above. This has been the source of a great deal of

TABLE 4.2. Different Types of Summaries

Session synopsis: A social worker at a rehabilitation facility is talking with two siblings about whether their mother should move back home or remain in a senior care center. Their mom recently broke her hip, and Medicare covered 2 weeks of postsurgical care. One sibling feels strongly about keeping their mom at home. The other sibling disagrees and favors the move to assisted living. The social worker thinks assisted living is more appropriate due to the mother's limited mobility and the home's layout.

Simple summary	"So, we've talked about your competing feelings about whether your mom should be here or go home. You have some financial concerns, and you think it would be money well spent. So, you two are going to hash it out and get back to me. Did I get everything?"
Brief refocusing	"Okay. So, you two both obviously care about your mom and want to do right by her. [Affirmation] You have some financial concerns about assisted living, uncertainty about whether her quality of life will be better here or at home, and strong feelings that families should care for their own. Could we turn our attention to talking more about what life here may be like for her?"
End of session	"So, today we talked about what to do with your mom. You both want the best for her but have different ideas about what that is. We talked about how moving her home may be challenging because her discharge date is tomorrow and the house may not be ready, and you have no services in place. You think she'd benefit from being here. However, you have some financial concerns and are willing to do the work to keep her at home, which includes setting up in-home services, getting a chair lift, so she can shower on the second floor, and rearranging the first floor to make it easier for her to move her walker. So, you're not quite sure which way to go yet and want to talk more about it now and get back to me."
Change talk	"You have some doubt, yet you can see how moving your mom may help her. You don't want her to be lonely, and you cannot be with her all the time. You liked the idea of her interacting with other seniors in rec groups. You also talked about how that would also reduce your stress with caretaking and would help you focus more on your teenage kids at home. It's like you're burning the candle at both ends. So, all in all, you're kind of leaning toward doing this. Of course, this decision is up to you because we can't make it for you. So, what do you think you'll do?"

confusion in the field about MI and may have prematurely led some helpers to think that they have already mastered it.

What distinguishes MI from more generalist counseling approaches that have some degree of training in these so-called active listening skills is the degree of skill and intentionality with which they are used. In MI, ROARS skills are used to deepen the sense of the MI Spirit experienced by family members and to also strategically work on resolving family members' ambivalence about behavior change or growth. In the next chapter, I further elaborate on how masterful use of these skills could lead to family members literally talking themselves into change.

CHAPTER 5

Working with Ambivalence

> Change, like sunshine, can be a friend or foe,
> a blessing or a curse, a dawn or a dusk.
> —WILLIAM ARTHUR WARD

Family members may be reluctant to engage in treatment. Or, during treatment, they may dig in their heels when asked to make certain changes. Family members worry that their loved one's failure to change could have catastrophic consequences, so they press harder for change. Pressing harder seems to go nowhere. Arguments ensue. One side argues for why a family member should change, and that person defends their position. How do we explain this reluctance to change when a problem seems obvious to us? This phenomenon goes by several terms, including impasse, disengagement, resistance, and denial.

In MI, we attribute some of these situations to ambivalence about decisions to change. Ambivalence involves mixed feelings or seeing both sides of the change equation. It accounts for both reasons for and against making behavior changes. And it is normal: Individuals will have mixed feelings when faced with a decision to make a change.

MI practitioners normalize, rather than demonize, ambivalence about behavior changes. The handling of ambivalence is one of the unique features of MI, distinguishing it from client-centered counseling and other approaches. This chapter reviews MI's conceptualization of ambivalence in detail, as well as strategies used to address it. Specifically, topics covered include:

1. Why the ambivalence concept is humanistic,
2. How to identify a target behavior,
3. How to recognize ambivalence toward changing a target behavior (i.e., change and sustain language),
4. How to evoke change language, and
5. How to progressively reinforce change language.

WHY CONCEPTUALIZE LACK OF CHANGE AS AMBIVALENCE?

Conceptualizing hesitancy about change as ambivalence is a deliberately bold and humanistic statement about the nature of change. Language shapes our attitudes and actions as helpers. For example, in my field, there is growing concern about using the term "substance abuse." Studies show that, when helpers viewing vignettes that describe individuals as "substance abusers," they expressed more punitive attitudes when compared to helpers seeing alternative vignettes (Kelly & Westerhoff, 2010). Some ways of describing substance use disorders also influence whether people think it is treatable (Kelly et al., 2021). In a similar vein, the language we use to conceptualize change processes has enormous potential to shape helpers' thoughts and actions when working with families.

Consider the implication of a helper telling a supervisor that a family is resistant to change. This may mean that there is a therapeutic impasse frustrating the helper. Yet, labeling a family as resistant, being in denial, or having low readiness to change may result in unfairly placing blame on families. There is a large difference between blaming a family for not changing and actively respecting their right to not change. A helper operating from the latter perspective proceeds with grace and acceptance, which can be communicated with the family. Perhaps change didn't occur in a given session, but the experience with the therapist was positive and accepting, increasing the chances for change or reengagement with services later. With MI, helpers often use the metaphor of planting seeds, recognizing that helping relationships may not meet everyone's expectations to start with, including the helpers'.

Language conventions about change may place blame on family members, also influencing helpers' interactions with them. A subtle look of disapproval or derisive statement may slip out, despite the helper's intention of developing rapport with all family members. Alternatively, a helper may simply lower their expectations for a family based on their attribution that a family is resistant to change. This may result in a self-fulfilling prophecy where their low expectations lead to poor outcomes. Expectations are important. We know family member expectations about change do influence actual change, but less research has been done on whether this is the case for clinicians' expectations about outcomes (Tambling, 2012). In summary, helpers' viewpoints on why families elect not to change are critical. They subtly influence interactions. Expecting ambivalence, and learning skills to resolve it, constitutes ethical practice.

Truly conceptualizing ambivalence as normal, and achieving full respect for family members' decisions not to change, may also be freeing for helpers. Anecdotally, some members of the MI community sense that growing their MI skills has helped them reduce compassion fatigue, a major problem in the helping field.[1] Thus, this conceptualization may help both family members and helpers alike. More research, however, is needed on whether utilizing MI reduces burnout among helpers.

> Expecting ambivalence, and learning skills to resolve it, constitutes ethical practice.

WHAT IS THE TARGET BEHAVIOR?

When thinking about whether one or more family members experience ambivalence, we first need to answer the question "What change is the family or family member ambivalent about making?" As noted earlier, this change is called the **target behavior**. It anchors how we look for signals of ambivalence and whether it is resolving or increasing.

In family work, target behaviors could include attending family sessions, completing tasks in between helping sessions, improving parenting, improving family communication, increasing affection, or decreasing conflict. Essentially, any clinical goal for the family may represent a target behavior. A target behavior is the object of ambivalence.

Defining a target behavior is an important first task when learning how to identify change and sustain language. Change talk and sustain talk, which we define below, serve as signals of ambivalence.

DETECTING AMBIVALENCE

Learning how to recognize ambivalence is the first step toward its resolution. As noted earlier, MI is talk therapy. Thus, we need to look for verbal

---

[1]However, one study randomized clinicians to an intervention or trained them in MI, measuring clinical burnout or intentions to leave the agency as clinician-level outcomes. Neither approach reduced burnout over time. See Salyers et al. (2019).

markers[2] of hesitancy or movement toward change. We understand these markers as part of change and sustain talk. Change talk is defined as a statement made by family members that indicates momentum toward change. On the other hand, sustain talk statements are ones made by family members that signal hesitancy.[3] One basic goal in MI is to increase the strength of change talk and empathically transition away from sustain talk.

> Aim to increase the strength of change talk and transition away from sustain talk.

Categories of Change and Sustain Talk

Several categories of change and sustain talk exist, forming the mnemonic DARN CAT: desire, ability, reasons, need, commitment, activation, and taking steps. In the sections that follow, I briefly define each category and give examples of change and sustain talk in each one. Table 5.1 presents an example of each type of change and sustain talk, all in reference to the same target behavior of improving family communication.

Desire

Desire is a strong word. Desire statements indicate what someone deeply wants. "I have been craving something like these exercises on fair fighting" is a strong example of a desire statement. "I wish things were different" is a somewhat weaker variant of a desire statement. Hence, some desire statements can be weaker than others. For example, the word "wish" may connote a more passive statement about change than the word "crave." The context of these statements also matters in thinking about the strength of change talk.

Ability

Ability, the next category of change talk, deals with the tools and confidence that the family member can muster. Ability overlaps with the concept of self-efficacy, or the belief that one can effect change easily. "I can do that" is a change talk statement that shows confidence about change.

---

[2] However, nonverbal behaviors such as facial expressions or silence can be interpreted as sustain-type behaviors and treated as such (e.g., "You're quiet today. I wonder if that means you're wondering if anything good will come out of this.").

[3] Change talk and change language are synonymous terms, as are sustain talk and sustain language. Thus, I will use them interchangeably throughout this book.

TABLE 5.1. That DARN CAT: Illustrative Examples of Change Talk and Sustain Talk for the Target Behavior of Improving Family Communication

	Change talk	Sustain talk
Desire	"That makes sense. I want to change how we talk about things."	"That's stupid. I don't want to change how we talk about things."
Ability	"We can take time to practice 'I statements.'"	"I'm no good with words." "This is gonna be hard."
Reasons	"If we improve our communication, we'll be less tense."	"Nothing good will come out of talking like this to each other."
Need	"Something has to change. We're nasty to each other."	"Nothing's wrong with our family's communication."
Commitment	"We will say nice things to each other every day this week."	"We are never going to try that."
Activation	"I'm willing to spend some time working on writing how I feel, so I have the words to practice 'I statements' when the conversations come up."	"Writing things down in advance of these real conversations is not something I'm willing to do. Seems a bit much."
Taking steps	"We did it. They said something nice to me every day, and I've really been working on 'I statements.'"	"We had a rough week. We weren't able to really practice 'I statements' this week."

Alternatively, "I am not sure I can do this" is an example of sustain talk showing low confidence to change. There are innumerable examples of this ability, including answers to a **scaling question** indicating high or low confidence in change, comments about hopelessness, or statements on how past successes give clients hope about their change efforts.

To illustrate the use of scaling questions in evoking change talk about one's ability to change, consider the following brief dialogue:

HELPER: And on a scale ranging from 0 to 10, where 0 is "not confident at all" and 10 is "completely confident," where would you put yourself? [Scaling question]

CLIENT: Maybe a 4 or a 5.

HELPER: And why are you a 4 or 5 and not a 0? [Open question]

CLIENT: (*Hesitates while thinking.*) Because, although I know it will be hard, I know I can do it if I make the decision to. I'm pretty good at sticking with my decisions.

HELPER: You're the type of person who sees things through. It's one of your strengths as a person. And your dilemma now is really deciding if the change is worth making. [Affirmation and reflection]

In this example, the part where the client said " . . . I know I can do it if I make the decision to . . . " is change talk signaling that they think they are able to change. Any reply above zero to a scaling question indicates some belief that they can change, even if it is weak. Here, the helper steers the conversation back to the topic of the importance of the change (i.e., desire, need, reasons). The helper steered the conversation there because the client said that they are able to do it if they make the decision.

Reasons

Perhaps the most straightforward category, reasons are often verbally stated benefits or costs of change. There is a long tradition of studying reasons for change. In my work, I've looked at developmental differences in types of reasons for change between adolescents and emerging adults, finding that the latter, on average, have less social pressure to quit using substances (Smith et al., 2010). Many instruments measuring reasons for change are publicly available, and helpers can administer them during intake assessments (see Appendix.).

An example of a reason for change may be "If we communicate better, we'll have more fun and be less tense in our relationship." On the contrary, a statement like "I don't want to talk about this. Working on family communication brings up unpleasant and private things" is an example of sustain language in this category.

Need

For me, this category seems to overlap with desire and reasons. I usually listen for instances of need when an urgency to change is expressed, such as "Something's gotta give," or the family member specifically uses the word "need."

Commitment

Unlike reason, desire, or need statements, those in this category imply strong resolve toward behavior change. Statements are less hypothetical, and change may sound imminent. "I will" implies commitment. "I agree to say something nice to my spouse every day after work" is commitment language regarding that task, perhaps mapping onto the broader target behavior of improved family communication. "I'm never going to come see you witch doctors," however, sounds like commitment to the status quo. Thus, it constitutes sustain language in the commitment category.

Activation

Activation refers to willingness to do an action. It is just a little more tentative than commitment language. For example, a client may state, "I'm thinking through how I can go to treatment. I'm about to get my affairs in order to do that."

Taking Steps

Perhaps one of the easiest categories to recognize, this category refers to actions taken by family members in the very recent past that are in the direction of change. An example may be a statement such as "We've practiced our 'I statements' a few times since last week."

Special Issues when Listening for Change and Sustain Talk

Recognition versus Categorization

I provide this mnemonic DARN CAT only as a tool to facilitate the broader goal of being able to recognize change language for a specific purpose. That purpose is being able to evoke and reinforce it until ambivalence is resolved. That is the end goal when there are no ethical problems with resolving ambivalence.[4] So, if you are new to learning MI, I encourage you to remember the big picture. If you get too caught up in deciding whether what the family member said was about desire or reasons for change, you may delay focus on the critical task of learning how to gently manage sustain talk,

---

[4]Some decisions involving change, such as whether to get a divorce, ethically require that we do not pursue change language in a specific direction. In those situations, we adopt the perspective of equipoise, not privileging change talk over sustain talk. See Chapter 8 for further discussion.

strengthen change talk, and resolve ambivalence.[5] In the next two sections, I provide more detail on how we elicit and reinforce change language to resolve ambivalence.

Simultaneous Change and Sustain Language

Sometimes family members will say something containing elements of both change and sustain talk in a single breath. Consider the statement "I could work on my communication easily, but I just haven't forgiven them enough to want to do so." The first half of the statement indicates an ability to participate in activities to improve family communication. Thus, it is change talk surrounding ability, the first A in DARN CAT. However, the second half of the statement about forgiveness is sustain talk. It is a reason not to move forward, the R in DARN CAT.

In situations like these, the helper will often have to choose between a few options, including (1) setting aside the change talk for a moment to empathize with the client, (2) focusing more on drawing out the change talk and placing less emphasis on the sustain talk, or (3) trying to address both simultaneously with a multipurpose statement. Below are three brief examples of how this may look.

Example 1: Empathy, Setting Aside Change Talk

FAMILY MEMBER: I could work on my communication, but I just haven't forgiven them enough to want to do so.

HELPER: You've been so hurt and want to talk more about forgiveness.

Example 2: Change Talk on Communication, with Low Empathy

FAMILY MEMBER: I could work on my communication easily, but I just haven't forgiven them enough to want to do so.

HELPER: You are confident that you could do these communication activities at home.

Example 3: Multipurpose Statement on Empathy and Change Talk

FAMILY MEMBER: I could work on my communication easily, but I just haven't forgiven them enough to want to do so.

---

[5] However, I have found knowing these categories to be helpful in supervision discussions. They provide a platform for discussing MI competency with our colleagues and supervisees when it comes to skill identifying change and sustain statements.

HELPER: Work on forgiveness may eventually open doors to better communication, and starting at forgiveness seems to make the most sense to you.

Statements containing both sustain and change language compel helpers to make decisions about what to emphasize. Above you can see several options for leaning more toward the MI Spirit dimension of empathy (1), the evocation of change talk only about ability (2), or a bit of both (3). This example leads us to an important topic of how we should progressively shift away from sustain language toward more change language to facilitate actual behavior change.

Transitioning from Sustain Language toward Evoking Change Talk

When family members are highly ambivalent about change, helpers are likely to hear much sustain language. When this is the case, it is critical to remember a couple of major principles. First and foremost, remember to maintain the accepting and empathic atmosphere while also focusing your attention on shifting from sustain to change language. Second, start with more tentative language when evoking change language.

Following these principles is critical. Imagine an archeological dig unearthing something invaluable and precious. Anyone can see the difference between using a spade versus wielding a small hand tool and gentle brush. The former goes deep fast but risks breaking what lies beneath. Spades use blunt force when breaking ground. **Use a brush, not a spade.** Alternatively, the latter approach of using a hand tool and gentle dusting brush exposes the treasure gently and precisely, minimizing damage. So, it is when helpers address change and sustain talk.

Balancing Acceptance and Empathy with Evocation

A difficult aspect of learning MI is developing the skill of deciding when to start working on change talk. Helpers I train often think of needing a full session or two (or more) just to build rapport with clients. Thus, for time-saving purposes, I argue that you can balance empathy and evocation of change talk. The key is mastering what I call multipurpose statements. Please briefly review Example 3 in the prior section again. In my estimation, that response communicates empathy and highlights the benefits of change. Thus, it would be both evocative and empathic, serving two purposes.

Using Tentative Language

When attempting to evoke change talk, wording matters. Helpers should try progressively and gently nudging toward increased change language, but it is easy to overshoot. If family members still express high levels of ambivalence, it may be important to add qualifying language to reflections such as "if you were to change," "you're considering," "you're starting to think that," or "a tiny bit." This is by no means an exhaustive list of qualifying language.

Remember not to be aggressive with your attempts to elicit or reinforce change talk. Consider the example of using a strongly worded statement like "You're really ready to change" right after the first signs of any blossoming change talk, when ambivalence is still rampant. Jumping right in like that would likely sacrifice empathy. Remember that empathy is a helper's ability to see the family member's perspective and accurately communicate it back to them. Thus, overshooting with too bold of an evocative reflection, for the purposes of generating change talk, may have the unintentional byproduct of lowering empathy. In other words, being empathic means that you can walk in a client's shoes in terms of accurately understanding their hesitations and motivations for change. By adding qualifiers, helpers can generate high-quality multipurpose statements, boosting both change talk and empathy. In summary, accurately recognizing the strength of change and sustain talk, and responding in kind, is part of being empathic.

One way to balance the tasks of communicating empathy and eliciting change talk involves using **double-sided reflections**. Double-sided reflections touch on both sides of the ambivalence, the change and the sustain talk. Consider the example of working with a youth who enjoys the sensations from using cannabis but is experiencing cannabis hyperemesis, severe cyclical vomiting due to use. Here, it would be easy for the clinician to solely focus on the negative aspect of using cannabis, the hyperemesis. Yet, overemphasis on the vomiting, while the youth still appears ambivalent, would lessen empathy. So, a double-sided reflection that may be useful in this situation would be "You're getting some benefits from weed and are also starting to worry about the increased vomiting." Double-sided reflections are multipurpose statements. They communicate empathy about sustain language while simultaneously eliciting change talk.

Strategies for Eliciting Change Talk

Table 5.2 shows a number of strategies that are used for eliciting change talk. They are the very micro-counseling skills reviewed in Chapter 4, but

TABLE 5.2. Strategies for Eliciting Different Types of Change Talk

DARN (desire, ability, reasons, need)

Strategies for eliciting	Examples	Type
[*Reflection*] "This sounds like something you think you need to do for your marriage."	"I gotta do something. It would kill me if we got divorced."	Desire
[*Reflection*] "You're quite sure this is going to be easy."	"Yeah. I could check his homework before 8 P.M. when I check out for the night."	Ability
[*Confidence ruler*] "On a scale of 1 to 10, how confident are you that you could make this change? Why are you a (enter client response) and not a 0?"	"A 6. We worked on communication before and things were good for a while."	Ability
[*Open question*] "What makes this the right time to make this change?"	"My mom would be happier with me, and things would be less tense."	Reasons
[*Importance ruler*] "On a scale of 1 to 10, how vital is it to make this change? Why are you a (client response) and not a 0?"	"A 3. I think I may need to talk to him."	Need
[*Amplified reflection*] "There really is no reason for you to join your family in these sessions."	"I don't know if I'd go that far. We definitely need something to change."	Need

CAT (commitment, activation, taking steps)

Strategies for eliciting	Examples	Type
[*Reflection*] "You'll do just about anything."	"Yeah, I'll see this through."	Commitment
[*Open question*] "What do you intend to do?"	"I plan to look into addressing my anger, so I don't take it out on them."	Activation
[*Open question*] "What is one small thing the three of you could do this week?"	"We could do something fun together to take our minds off all these problems. It's been all negative lately."	Taking steps
[*Reflection*] "You're ready to try some new things, and now you want to define what those things are."	"We just sat down and mapped out a schedule, so we know who would be giving her the medication at what times."	Taking steps

here they're being used intentionally for evoking change talk. This is by no means an exhaustive list of useful reflections, open questions, or readiness rulers/scaling questions; rather, it illustrates the general principle of how these skills can be used to evoke change talk.

Remember, these micro-counseling skills can be used for other purposes besides generating change talk. Consider the simple paraphrase "Okay, so you came in today because you have been having some issues with mistrust in your relationship." This is a perfectly good reflection for summarizing what the client just said and communicating that you are listening. It also perhaps encourages the family members to say more about mistrust by emphasizing it in the reflection. However, it is not yet evoking what we refer to above as change talk. Consider the alternative statement "So you came in today to work on mistrust issues and seem pretty eager to get started on this." That bit at the end about eagerness is a little added emphasis that converts a simple paraphrase into a reflection with potential to evoke change talk from the family members.

Although this example was specifically about increasing a reflection's potential to elicit change talk, the same principle applies to all the other ROARS skills defined in Chapter 4. For example, open questions can be used for history taking, such as asking, "What do you like to do for fun as a family?" Conversely, helpers can design open questions to ask directly for change talk, such as "How did you conclude that coming to see someone like me was a good idea?" This open question is specifically asking for a reason for seeking treatment, which, when answered, would constitute change talk in the reason category described earlier.

Inferring Motivation

Family members may not explicitly say what factors motivate them to change. However, they will drop a lot of clues that can be massaged into actual client change talk. Just showing up to a session, for example, constitutes some degree of motivation. Consider an initial session wherein a family member voices outright that they are not happy about seeking a family helper. This begs the question of why they even walked through the door. Yet, that action presumes some level of motivation. A frequently used reflection in response to a bold statement about not wanting to be in a session, while also sitting there, is "You have reservations, and yet you came. Tell me what's in this for you and why you came today." This is another example of a double-sided reflection, which here is followed by an open question.

Listen for clues that can be massaged into change talk.

Helpers can view family members' statements from either a glass-half-full or glass-half-empty perspective. For example, I recall a situation in my substance use treatment work where a client voiced a desire to go get drunk one last time before starting treatment. That could (rightly so) be viewed as a highly negative behavior, raising concerns.[6] Alternatively, a helper could interpret this comment as a precursor to change talk. Getting drunk one last time appears like an unconventional step to take en route to behavior change, but perhaps it is normal for this individual. A reflection that may help frame this as potential change talk could be "This last hoorah is part of you saying goodbye to alcohol, and you are ready to go to treatment." Here, motivation is inferred from the second part of the reflection. Be on the lookout for statements that at first glance seem problematic but for which you may infer family members' motivations for change.

SPOTLIGHTING CHANGE TALK

MI seeks to resolve ambivalence by progressively reinforcing change talk. Here, reinforcement is a fancy word for spotlighting change talk while using the momentum of the change talk to guide the discussion toward a decision about change or articulation of an action plan.

Like evoking change talk, helpers reinforce change talk with the ROARS skills discussed in Chapter 4. Table 5.3 gives examples of how to reinforce change talk. Remember, when discussing the reinforcement of change talk, we are examining what the helper should say after a family member's change talk. Thus, Table 5.3 shows the family member statement prompting the helper's reinforcing statement.

Additionally, the same principle of using tentative language and not overshooting family members' statements applies to reinforcing change talk. There are some nuances to reinforcing change talk in the sections that follow. These include (1) deciding when to focus on resolving ambivalence and when to shift the focus of the conversation away from it, (2) remembering that for some target behaviors it is not ethical to progressively reinforce change talk toward a particular decision, (3) troubleshooting what to do when you hear redundant change talk, and (4) shifting from motivation to action.

---

[6] Directly telling a client not to get drunk one last time before entering treatment may violate client autonomy, one dimension of the MI Spirit. However, there are autonomy-enhancing ways you can express concerns. The steps involved are asking for permission to share a concern, sharing it, and using an open question to assess the client's reaction about the concern. Be genuine. If it is hard for you to see value in reflecting like this example, consider expressing your concern in a way that enhances autonomy.

TABLE 5.3. Strategies for Spotlighting Different Types of Change Talk

DARN (desire, ability, reasons, need)

Type of change talk	Examples	Reinforcing change talk (used after change talk)
Desires	"I really need to be more present with my family."	"Tell me why it would be a good thing for you to be more 'present.'" [Elaboration through open question]
Ability	"I could start backing up my partner when she sets a consequence."	"You're confident you can do this and see it helping with the family." [Reflection]
Reasons	"I want to get a job, and my mom would be happier with me, and I may think more clearly."	"You have lots of reasons for cutting back on marijuana. You want to get back to work, may see some improvements with your relationship with your mom, and you're excited [*added emphasis here to make complex*] about the possibility of thinking more clearly. So, what are the next steps for you?" [Summary]
Need	"I have to do right by my mom."	"How will making this change make things better for your mom?" [Elaboration]

CAT (commitment, activation, taking steps)

Type of change talk	Examples	EARS skills (used after change talk)
Commitment	"I will do whatever it takes."	"I think it is outstanding that you are so committed to changing with your family." [Affirmation]
Activation	"Maybe you could help me plan out how to ask my dad to be less critical of me."	"You're ready to take that step . . . figuring out how to say it to him, so it sticks. You think this will help you spur some change in him or, if it doesn't work, just give you the dignity in knowing you did it."
Taking steps	"Things aren't perfect, but I've been doing some of the things we talked about last time."	"You're trying hard. You want your family life to be better. Now, it's all about tinkering with what will work best for you." [Reflection]

Spotlighting Requires Focus

In MI conversations, there can exist a large degree of focus on spotlighting change talk, temporarily at the expense of exploring topics other than resolving ambivalence for a target behavior. Thus, the progressive reinforcement aspect of MI is best used when there is a clear target behavior for which ambivalence exists. This aspect of MI is not designed for the goal of broad exploration of all clinical issues experienced by the family. When spotlighting change talk, information often surfaces that clinicians want to explore as naturally curious helpers.

Sometimes information comes up that helpers feel compelled to address on the spot. Consider the parent who says they want to learn better parenting strategies to stop an intergenerational cycle of violence within their family.[7] Here, the target behavior is improving parenting, as there was ambivalence about attending parenting classes. The helper could proceed with spotlighting the change talk or could feel tempted to shift gears and explore the family's past experience of violence. By exploring the past, the helper would step away from progressively focusing on change language and the goal of resolving ambivalence about the referral to parenting classes.

Making these decisions about whether to stay the course with MI to resolve ambivalence or change course to a new topic is often difficult to do in real time. First, there is an issue of safety, as well as required legal obligations should issues of abuse or neglect come up. Second, helpers must ask themselves what gains occur if the topic shifts. Is it better to resolve ambivalence about the behavior change, or would changing topics lead to better rapport or new directions? Sometimes this decision also depends on where in the therapeutic process you are—early or late sessions—with a specific family member. If you are still working on engagement and resolving ambivalence about session attendance, perhaps staying the course on change talk about that target behavior takes priority. You cannot thoroughly address other topics if clients do not come back. Attendance may be particularly problematic if you open up traumatic topics too fast. Finally, consider what you know about yourself as a helper. Are you a naturally curious person who tends to get distracted easily? Do your sessions seem to meander? Do you really need to know the information you seek? Do you need that information right now?

---

[7]This example comes from a video I frequently use in training. A full video with a transcript is available. See the "My father also hit me" resource in the Appendix.

Ethical Issues with Reinforcing Change Talk

One other caveat about change talk: Remember to use your powers for good. You should be asking yourself if MI is appropriate for some target behaviors. Remember that sometimes it may be unethical to have clients talk themselves into change, and this situation calls for maintaining **equipoise**, meaning equal weighting of change and sustain talk in reference to a decision. I previously noted that we should not use MI to have family members talk themselves into getting a divorce. Reinforcing pro-divorce statements (e.g., "If you left, you'd be free to pursue what you really want in life") and trying to tip the balance in that direction is not ethical practice.

Many helpers use a **decisional balance exercise** where family members write down the pros and cons of a specific decision. Miller and Rollnick (2023) provide an excellent template that can be used in practice, where a client considers (1) the advantages of change (i.e., change talk), (2) the advantages of not changing (i.e., sustain talk), (3) the disadvantages of change (i.e., sustain talk), and (4) the disadvantages of not changing (i.e., change talk).

When doing decisional balance exercises with family members, completely neutral discussion and autonomy respect are key (see the box below). Clients decide the next course of action. A helper imposing their agenda by highlighting one side or another of the ledger would violate the principle of respecting family members' autonomy.

Decisional Balance to Maintain Equipoise

Decisional balance activities are used when there are ethical reasons to not sway an ambivalent person toward a choice (Miller & Rollnick, 2009, 2023). There is some confusion about whether decisional balance is part of MI or not. For example, some studies on MI use decisional balance even when they are clearly trying to influence participants toward a change (e.g., reduce substance use). Furthermore, in earlier writings, Miller and Rollnick (2009) explicitly said that MI was not to be conflated with decisional balance-based treatments. Given this, and findings showing that decisional balance exercises do not resolve ambivalence (Miller & Rose, 2015), it is not surprising that this confusion exists. Simply put, it is currently recommended to emphasize change talk in MI when it can be done ethically. Decisional balance activities are used when helpers want to maintain equipoise.

Redundant Change Talk?

New learners of MI may have the tendency to evoke one single reason for change, to keep circling back to that reason, and to call it quits with evocation and reinforcement of change talk. That is not ideal. Building motivation through progressive reinforcement of change talk takes some effort and time. This reinforcement may be the sole focus of a significant portion of a session or couple of sessions for a single target behavior.

What should be done if the three different techniques are used for evoking change talk (e.g., scaling question, open question, and reflection) and the family member only lists one single type of change talk (i.e., desire, ability, reason, need, commitment, activation, taking steps)? Typically, when I'm presented with this scenario, there are a few considerations worth mentioning. First, has the helper mastered reflections and complex reflections? These skills become critical in the process of reinforcing change talk. Second, how well is the clinician doing at recognizing change talk or clues about motivation when it is implicit and needs to be drawn out. Third, a lack of breadth in change talk may indicate that the helper wants to move at a quicker pace than the family member, perhaps prematurely rushing to solutions. Finally, if the change talk is really strong, it may be that the family member is not experiencing significant ambivalence. In this situation, briefer reinforcement and transitioning to discussion of action planning may be indicated. Remember, MI is intended to address ambivalence.

Transitioning toward Action Planning

A family member has told their helper all the reasons they have for improving their communication, change talk was reinforced, and it seems like the session has reached a turning point. There seems to be a recognized need for change, and things seem a little lighter or less tense. But how exactly should the helper proceed? Now what?

Often, the question "So, what do you think you'll do?" bridges the gap between the why and the how of change. This is sometimes referred to as the **key question** in MI. Like all MI micro-counseling skills, this one is not foolproof, but it does seem useful in prompting the articulation of action steps.

Reflections can also be used to nudge toward the expression of action steps. For example, consider the reflection "You're starting to see some potential benefits to coming to a place like this and now are beginning to think through next steps." In reflections, it seems like the small clause "and now" queues family members to think forward and nudges on verbalizing activities.

SUMMARY

This chapter introduced readers to the core concepts of evoking and reinforcing change talk, the central mechanism in MI that aids in resolving ambivalence about behavior change. Some key principles include being tentative in one's responses, remaining empathic and accepting while keeping an eye out for change and sustain language, and working toward progressive reinforcement of change language.

As these skills can be used at multiple times throughout the course of the therapeutic relationship, subsequent chapters will elaborate on sequencing. In the chapters that follow, I address using these skills during various tasks of treatment, such as engagement, focusing, and terminating services. I also expand on conceptual issues of evoking and reinforcing change talk when target behaviors occur at the family level, as well as when helpers are conducting conjoint sessions.

PART II

USING MOTIVATIONAL INTERVIEWING WITH FAMILIES

CHAPTER 6

Moving toward Integration of Motivational Interviewing and Family Work

> If you cannot get rid of the family skeleton, you may as well make it dance.[1]
> —George Bernard Shaw

> Home is where you are loved the most and act the worst.
> —Marjorie Pay Hinckley

In Chapter 1, I defined *family-centered care* broadly as any service in which one or more members of a client's intimate social network encounters a helper, either together or separately. Given this broad definition, it is impossible to do a comprehensive review of all major schools of family therapy or even every possible type of family work. Remember, too, that family work is far from limited to formal family therapy. So, this chapter focuses on how MI is compatible with different family therapy models. I introduce some overarching concepts such as systems theory, the family life cycle, and homeostasis. Then, I briefly review major models of family therapy, highlighting places where MI and family work have synergy.

KEY CONCEPTS IN FAMILY WORK

Families Are Systems

The *sine qua non* of family work is acknowledging the importance of broader systems on individual behavior. In their seminal work in the 1950s,

---

[1] With an acknowledgment to The Society of Authors on behalf of the Bernard Shaw Estate.

Gregory Bateson and his colleagues applied the biologically oriented systems theory plus a separate theory of human–machine interaction, called cybernetics, to families. Carr (2015) calls their work both revolutionary and paradigm-shifting because, for the first time, pathology was conceptualized in terms of interpersonal interactions. This was as revolutionary an idea as conceptualizing resistance in terms of interpersonal interactions in MI, which I discuss in the section that follows.

In the systemic view, family members' interactions with each other form feedback loops, which have the power to reinforce certain behaviors. For example, let's say that a child's sarcastic remarks prompt their parent to raise their voice. This yelling, in turn, causes the child to withdraw to their room, feeling deflated and inconsequential. Perhaps to reclaim a sense of control, as the child can predict their parent's response, they wield sarcasm again. The pattern persists uninterrupted as part of a broader family communication problem, leading to feeling distant from one another.

Family workers, by extension of this systems view, reframe problems for families in interactional terms and attempt to change such interactions. For example, a helper that meets this parent and child may be told this child has been diagnosed with oppositional defiant disorder (ODD), firmly locating the problem as being within the child (i.e., an identified client approach). In a family systems approach, however, the helper would work toward illuminating the very family interactions described above, trying to disrupt those that are stuck in predictable, negative patterns.

To give another example, family members often directly tell helpers how they feel about or what they want from other members. When these instances arise in session, helpers gradually begin to instruct family members to speak directly to each other. Often, this is a sign of progress in families that are too conflictual to have such conversations on their own without escalating into familiar conversational scripts. In essence, in vitro alteration of communication patterns is one example of working systemically with families. The goal of many systemic approaches to family work is to change the conversation, not to merely repeat these cyclical communication patterns in front of a helper.

Systems and MI

This focus on family systems is highly compatible with modern conceptualizations of how MI produces its salubrious effects. MI is a systems approach focused on interactions between helpers and family members. That is, just as family therapy focuses on interactions between various family members, voluminous MI process work exists that examines conversations between helpers and clients. In other words, MI concerns itself with the helper–client dyadic system.

To illustrate how many MI practitioners are already taking a systems approach, consider the notion connected with the MI approach: "Resistance is interpersonal." This saying epitomizes a systemic view on client motivation. A nonsystemic view on client motivation would place the locus of motivation inside the client, conceptualizing it as a personal attribute. Whenever I hear professional helpers say, "How do you work with unmotivated clients?" I instantly suspect they may be operating from a nonsystemic perspective on client motivation. So, just as family workers spend time with families on perceiving their problems systemically, MI trainers work with trainees on viewing the helping relationship and client motivation systemically.

To illustrate this principle of viewing MI as an application of systems theory to the helper–family member dyad, consider the following short dialogue where a feedback loop is established. You will hear a helper evoking sustain talk and then subsequently reinforcing it, calling into question whether the "resistance" is actually located in the family member, or if it is actually a product of the interaction at the systems level. Remember that, as discussed in Chapter 5, evoking and reinforcing sustain talk is the exact opposite of what we want to do clinically in the MI model. Doing this is thought to reinforce ambivalence.

PARENT: He has oppositional defiant disorder. I'm not able to get through to him, and it's making my life miserable.

HELPER: That must be hard for you. But to be honest, I don't really believe in ODD. For me, I think it's a bit overdiagnosed. [Confrontation]

PARENT: I guess we'll just have to agree to disagree on that. He has all the classic symptoms, and his psychiatrist was pretty sure he has it. [Sustain talk]

HELPER: Well, one thing I'd like to work on here is focusing more on your interactions with him. It could be that you're doing some things that bring out his "symptoms." (*Helper uses fingers to make air quotes.*) I can help with that. [Advising without permission]

PARENT: Are you really blaming me for his diagnosis?

In this short exchange, there was ambivalence by the parent about whether to conceptualize the problem as an individual or family problem. Unfortunately, if you conceptualize the helper–client dyad as a system, you can see how this interaction serves to increase, rather than resolve, the parent's ambivalence. Imagine this helper later telling their supervisor that they tried to move this parent toward a systems perspective on their family problems, but the parent is resistant. It may present as ironic to someone well versed in MI that a helper is trying to impact a family system while ignoring the dynamics of the helper–family member dyadic system. By using a confrontational style, the helper activated the client's ambivalence and the parent offered sustain talk, which we described in Chapter 2 as a key factor that maintains ambivalence and oftentimes stalls behavior change.

Let's briefly look at a feedback loop that may help the client resolve any ambivalence about their role in maintaining family communication problems.

PARENT: He has oppositional defiant disorder. I'm not able to get through to him, and it's making my life miserable.

HELPER: That must be hard for you. You're not always sure how to respond to him when he's acting out. [Empathy, complex reflection]

PARENT: Exactly. I'm constantly walking on eggshells.

HELPER: You want your communication to improve and to feel more relaxed. [Evocative complex reflection]

PARENT: When he throws me a shit sandwich, I just choke. I either yell or say something snarky. He then just feeds off that.

HELPER: So, you see a pattern in how you talk to each other. You don't like how you respond, and then he escalates. You wish there were other ways. [Complex reflection] If I may, that's a lot of what family work is about. We provide the space for you two to try out new ways of talking to each other and look at ways to prevent you from having the same old conversation again and again. What are your thoughts on trying something like that? [Collaborative open question]

PARENT: That actually sounds really great.

These short examples illustrate two principles. First, they demonstrate how helpers pursuing family work try to shift family members' perspectives toward a systemic view of their problems. Second, they illustrate how the helper–client dyad can be considered a system and how interactions within this system can either maintain or promote the resolution of ambivalence.

In short, all family work builds on the premise that groups of people linked by tight biological or communal bonds influence each other. This influence is conceptualized as feedback within the family system. However, theoretical assumptions drive beliefs about where systems falter and need repairs. Thus, after discussing two additional transtheoretical concepts about family life cycles and homeostasis below, I then briefly examine some of the major theoretical models underpinning family work, highlighting opportunities for the integration of MI.

Family members influence each other.

Families in the Life Cycle

Here, I take a lifespan approach to families. In essence, this means that we should mind the major developmental tasks of various family members. Typically, families with young children, school-age children, adolescents, ready-to-launch children, and grown children face different, yet predictable, developmental dilemmas. Families commonly need help at transition points when stressors peak (McGoldrick & Shibusawa, 2012). Family life cycles are also highly varied, with Walsh (2012) arguing for the adoption of a "flexible family life cycle" heuristic. Thus, the family life cycle can coexist peacefully with the varied forms that families take (i.e., stepfamilies, nonmarried cohabiting couples, LGBTQ couples with adopted children, older parents of young children), and such an approach need not be limited to romanticized views of traditional nuclear families from the 1950s (Walsh, 2012).

Most accrediting bodies require health services to be developmentally appropriate. This is excruciatingly difficult to measure and define. In-depth knowledge of the family lifespan may result in helpers being able to show compassion and empathy for various family members. This, in turn, will lead to better outcomes. For example, if you are not a parent, can you imagine what it is like to be a middle-aged parent with a teenage child who suffers from a mental health condition? What does their life look like? Perhaps a parent has family troubles at both ends of the spectrum, as middle-aged individuals often have both child raising and elder care commitments. They may be struggling to balance work with family obligations and your time with them may be squeezed into their jam-packed schedule. Fortunately, to do MI well, you don't have to have the same lived experiences as your clients. Instead, having a general, albeit nonrigid, sense of how people experience family life during various ages may enable helpers to translate that knowledge into reflections (see Chapter 4). In other words, sometimes accurate empathy will involve recognizing family life cycle issues and translating them into effective reflective listening statements. Exercise 6.1 provides an activity for using life stage information in your reflections.

EXERCISE 6.1. Working toward Lifespan Accuracy in Your Reflections

Directions: This exercise is intended to help you use developmental information in reflections with people at various life stages. In the middle column, write what you know about that developmental stage. In the rightmost column, write how you may use that information in reflections used with a person in that life stage.

Lifespan information	Common developmental features/stressors?	What aspects of development could be rolled into reflections?
Example: 6-year-old transitioning to first grade	*Example:* Still learning abstract thinking skills.	*Example:* Knowledge of popular films or cartoons known to the child could be used in metaphor-style reflections. May aid in engagement and match concrete thinking style.
14-year-old transitioning to high school		
18-year-old transitioning to university		
25-year-old entering the workforce		
Person in their late 20s still living at home		
New parent in their early 30s		
Unmarried career-focused person in their 30s		
Unmarried person in their 40s with a disability who lives with older sibling		
New parent in their early 50s		
Middle-aged person caring for both their elderly parents and their teenage children		
Older person who is remarrying after death of a spouse		
Grandparent who is raising their grandchildren		

80

Homeostasis

A core concept used in most family work is **homeostasis**, or the tendency of the family system to maintain its balance. Families would indeed be chaotic if they remained in active conflict for long periods of time. So, they tend to develop communication patterns or structures to restore balance, stability, and predictability.

An application of the principle of homeostasis is that if one individual begins making changes in their behavior it will inevitably impact the family system. The family needs to adapt to behavior change to maintain order. Consider a family that for three hours a night watches television together in relative silence, with various family members also attached to other electronic devices such as smart phones or tablets. Yes, there is occasional family banter, but one member grows tired of this well-established family ritual. Now imagine that member of the family proudly announcing that they no longer wish to watch as much television at night. They cite boredom, a lack of feeling close to other members, and concerns about their weight. In this example, homeostasis could be maintained by the other members if they bond together against this defector to perpetuate their behavior (i.e., structural alliance). Or they may elect to simply not talk about it and go about their business with one family member going out more at night or reading silently in their room, while other family members continue on. The recent change in the nightly ritual must not be discussed or it would disrupt the family's homeostasis.

> **If one individual changes their behavior, it will impact the whole family system.**

Homeostasis is also linked with transition points in the family life cycle (Colapinto, 2016). For example, the equilibrium achieved by certain familial behavioral patterns may be disrupted when a new member leaves (i.e., death, divorce, child leaving for college) or enters the family (i.e., birth, remarriage). These flashpoints may create crises that require changes in one or more members of the family in order to restore balance.

So, one task for helpers to consider is what changes are perturbing the family system, and how the family attempts to maintain stability. Sharing observations with families about these patterns can be done in a manner consistent with MI, either through reflections or by asking permission to share an idea about how the family system is operating. However, confrontational or overly persuasive tactics to convince a family about how their family system is functioning are contraindicated in MI.

To effectively use MI with families, remain mindful of the concepts of systemic interactions, family life cycles, and homeostasis. The key task of integrating MI into family work is translating this knowledge into effective communication that helps build warm environments and shape family members' speech toward change.

MODELS OF FAMILY WORK

As noted, interest in family therapy waxed in the middle of the 20th century, in part due to psychodynamic and humanistic models that explicitly acknowledged the role of the family in individual functioning (Nichols & Davis, 2020). There are many different models of family therapy. The major schools of family therapy include systemic, structural, cognitive-behavioral, solution-focused, and ecological. The current trend is toward eclectic practice that is systemic in nature and focuses on general factors that promote change, which are also referred to as common factors (Sprenkle et al., 2009). Nevertheless, there is some value in learning the basic assumptions of the various schools of family therapy, as they have slightly different emphases that drive intervention targets.

What follows is a brief overview of select models, including structural family therapy, cognitive-behavioral family therapy, solution-focused family therapy, and ecological family therapy. Because systemic family therapy principles cut across all these models, and I have already laid out the general principles of family systems theory, I won't review this model further. Nichols and Davis (2020) provide a more comprehensive, yet accessible treatment of all major schools of family therapy. Here, I provide a short history of each model, discuss how they conceptualize problems and change targets, and briefly review the main techniques. Then, I discuss opportunities and challenges for blending MI with each model.

Structural Family Therapy

Structural family therapy was developed in the 1970s by Salvador Minuchin (1974) and colleagues at the Minuchin Center for the Family, an influential training center for family therapists (Nichols &Davis, 2020). Because the originator was a child psychiatrist, this model is mainly used with families with children (Colapinto, 2016). As Minuchin himself emphasized later in his career, contemporary models of structural family therapy emphasize broader ecological systems in which families are nested. Such models are efficacious at reducing substance use and other conduct problems in adolescents (Baldwin et al., 2012).

Structural family therapists eye the hierarchies and patterns of interactions within families. They particularly watch for loose or rigid boundaries such as problematic cross-generational alliances (e.g., father and son gang up on mother), mapping deeply ingrained communication patterns onto problems. Minuchin (1974) believed that many family problems were ordinary problems of living that peaked when there was a mismatch between the family structure and a developmental transition. For example, parents could scapegoat a child's problems when in fact there was a problem with the marital subsystem, one structure within the broader set of family structures. Thus, the scapegoating served the purpose of conflict avoidance and maintaining homeostasis. Conversely, enmeshment or disengagement may exist, also resulting in problems. Behaviors are explained in terms of the structures involved. For example, a parent tries to discipline a child and their partner rebukes this effort in front of the child. The parent, angered by their failed discipline effort, then recedes into their bedroom, withdrawing from the other partner and child. This pattern would be conceptualized by a structural family therapist as a problem with boundaries between two structures, the parental and child subsystems. This model seeks to restructure the family, as problems are conceptually linked to boundaries in the family hierarchy and resulting communication patterns.

Therapeutic Techniques

Major techniques used to restructure family interactions include joining, reframing, enactment, and unbalancing. Joining means that the helper enters the family system, as if they are a family member and part of the system itself. In some instances, the helper will sit between two enmeshed family members if their alliance needs restructuring (e.g., weak parent subsystem and strong parent–child alliance). Reframing refers to the process of conceptualizing problems as family and interactional problems versus individual problems. For example, if a family member refers to the symptomatic person in the family, the helper may correct them by saying that the problem is a family and not an individual problem. Enactment is the process where helpers ask the family to discuss the problem as they normally do at home, for the purpose of getting a sense of their communication patterns and the structure of the family. This technique may reveal repeated patterns of communication and unhealthy alliances. Finally, unbalancing is a highly directive strategy that consists of the helper temporarily siding with one party in the family for the express purpose of rearranging the family structure. Though it is beyond the scope of this chapter, Colapinto (1982, 2016) provides an excellent summary of these strategies with case examples.

Opportunities for Integration of MI

Two major similarities between MI and structural family therapy render them good bedfellows. First, both are active treatments that rely on intensive observation of clients. In MI, helpers listen with a keen ear for the purpose of delivering accurate reflection statements that convey empathy and resolve ambivalence. In structural family therapy, helpers examine how families talk about problems and observe for specific patterns of communications that may signify the presence of enmeshment, disengagement, scapegoating, or other intervention targets that are dealt with in real time during sessions. In fact, cases replete with examples of high-quality reflective listening appear in Minuchin's (1974) seminal work describing structural family therapy. Furthermore, both models concern themselves with assessment in the here and now. Ambivalence in MI is conceptualized as a current problem, as are family interactions that may need altering. Thus, excessive history taking is deemphasized in both models.

MI and structural family therapy make good bedfellows.

Yet, there are likely places in structural family therapy where the underlying MI Spirit can be followed more closely. For example, by Colapinto's (1982) account some structural family therapists employ more directive and confrontational approaches than others. Direct confrontation in MI is contraindicated given the emphasis on how client ambivalence that is met with one-sided confrontation results in further impasse. So, if a family member balks at a restructuring attempt, it likely signals ambivalence, for which MI is well suited.

Cognitive-Behavioral Family Therapy

Based in the learning principles, cognitive-behavioral family therapy generally uses the language of reinforcement and punishment, while simultaneously recognizing the role of cognition in behavior. Thus, behaviors that are reinforced continue, while those that are punished or ignored can ultimately be extinguished. Even small steps toward the desired behavior, or approximations, are reinforced to shape behavior toward the fully desired behavior. Although classic learning theory focused mainly on stimulus and response patterns, cognitive theorists emphasized the intermediary role of thoughts. Regarding cognitions, initially individualistic concepts such as negative self-talk (Beck et al., 1979) were eventually expanded to include cognitions about interpersonal relationships. For example, family members may make up their own stories they tell themselves, whether accurate or not, to explain their family member's behavior (Karney & Bradbury, 2000). Such stories may make inaccurate assumptions about how the other party is thinking or why they acted a certain way. These assumptions, such as continually assuming hostile intent on the part of one's family member(s), can result in the maintenance of communication problems and distress.

Another theoretical influence undergirding cognitive-behavioral family therapy is Bandura's (1977) social learning theory. Social learning states that through observation, people learn skills and increase their confidence, or self-efficacy, in enacting new behaviors. This theory is the bedrock for many CBT-oriented techniques involving modeling new behaviors and skills that may help families address their current problems.

Therapeutic Techniques

Cognitive-behavioral practitioners emphasize concrete and teachable skills and emphasize the setting of SMART goals. SMART is a mnemonic for specific, measurable, achievable, realistic, and time-limited. Thus, cognitive-behavioral family therapy is typically a time-limited therapeutic approach relative to insight-oriented therapies such as psychodynamic models, which are generally long-lasting treatments. Select examples of cognitive-behavioral family therapy models with excellent empirical support include Patterson's parent training model (Forgatch & Patterson, 2010), behavioral couples therapy (Epstein & McCrady, 1998; O'Farrell & Fals-Stewart, 2012), the community reinforcement approach with family training (Smith & Meyers, 2007), and the adolescent community reinforcement approach (Godley et al., 2016).

Other techniques in cognitive-behavioral family therapy include cognitive restructuring (Dattilio, 2005) and assigning homework to complete between sessions. Cognitive restructuring in the family context involves attempting to shift family members' perceptions of each other's motives or behaviors. Regrettably, although restructuring is supported as a mechanism of change for cognitive-behavioral therapy in individual treatments for mood disorders (Kazantzis et al., 2018), it is unclear if restructuring is an active ingredient in cognitive-behavioral family therapy. For example, there were no differences in clinical outcomes of distressed couples who received versions of CBT-based family therapy with or without restructuring (Baucom et al., 1990). Godley et al.'s (2016) adolescent community reinforcement approach provides families with a daily reminder to be nice to attempt to increase self-monitoring of positive communication behaviors.

Opportunities for Integration with MI

Most applications of MI involve resolving ambivalence for behavior change in very time-limited treatment approaches. Furthermore, we know little about using MI in later stages of family work. For example, motivational enhancement therapy in project MATCH, one of the largest ever studies of alcohol use disorder treatment, lasted only four sessions. Similarly, in the largest study of the treatment of adolescent outpatient cannabis use disorders, MI was paired with five or 12 sessions of cognitive-behavioral therapy. It is no surprise that motivation is considered essential for treatment engagement. Note that in these models that involved MI, it was not adapted for use with the whole family system, but rather targeted at the individual presenting for treatment.

Additionally, these MI protocols were short and were frontloaded in the treatment protocols. So, we know very little about using MI in later stages of the cognitive-behavioral family treatments. It seems, however, that ambivalence can materialize at any stage of the helping relationship. For example, what if a family member balks at a particular homework assignment during the middle of treatment? Additionally, could MI be used later in cognitive-behavioral-based family therapies to consolidate commitments to continue practicing skills use after termination? We will explore some of these topics in subsequent chapters on the four tasks of MI: engaging, focusing, evoking, and planning. Readers interested in learning more on the integration of MI and CBT can refer to Naar and Safren's (2017) comprehensive coverage of this topic.

Solution-Focused Family Therapy

Initially developed by Insoo Kim Berg and Steven de Shazer in the late 1980s and 1990s, solution-focused therapy is currently very popular (Berg, 1994; de Shazer, 1988; Nichols & Davis, 2020). It is a brief therapy model premised on the idea that people have solutions to their own problems but get overwhelmed and stuck. This premise overlaps substantially with MI's conceptualization of ambivalence. That is, just as solution-focused helpers try to evoke solutions from family members, helpers using MI try to evoke change talk, one form of which involves solutions to problems (e.g., activation and taking steps). At face value, solution-focused therapy also shares much in common with cognitive-behavioral therapy in terms of being a short-term and action-oriented approach that emphasizes concrete and achievable goals.

Consistent with the model's here-and-now view of therapy, solution-focused therapy's originators wrote little about theoretical orientation. In fact, de Shazer and Dolan (2012) wrote, "SFBT [solution-focused brief therapy] is not theory based but was pragmatically developed. One can clearly see the roots of SFBT in the early work of the Mental Research Institute in Palo Alto and of Milton H. Erickson; in Wittgensteinian philosophy; and in Buddhist thought" (p. 1). Instead, solution-focused therapy operates under some plain language assumptions, such as the following: (1) If it isn't broken, don't fix it; (2) If something works, do more of that; (3) If it is not working, do something different; (4) There are always exceptions to when problems occur which yield clues about what to do differently; (5) Talking about problems is different from talking about solutions; (6) Small steps can lead to big changes; and (7) The solution is not directly related to the problem (de Shazer & Dolan, 2012).

Solution-focused therapy enjoys tremendous popularity with social workers, who have been highly influenced by an emphasis of focusing on client strengths rather than problems (Saleebey, 2012). It also seems to share a lot in common with evolving clinical applications of positive psychology, based on the seminal work of researchers who emphasized studying the promotion of happiness, rather than the elimination of pathology (Diener, 1984).

Therapeutic Techniques

Similar to MI's emphasis on evoking change talk, helpers using solution-focused therapy try to evoke language about exceptions to problem occurrence, as well as language surrounding what clients will be doing differently when the presenting problem is no longer raging. For example, helpers will ask exception-finding questions such as "In thinking about times this has not been a problem for you, what were you doing differently?" This is typically followed by recommendations to do more of that (i.e., "do more of what works" principle). The main techniques in SFT include scaling questions, exception finding questions, and use of the miracle question.

Opportunities for Integration with MI

Much overlap exists between solution-focused therapy and MI techniques. Both emphasize a particular use of language. Whereas solution-focused therapy attempts to avoid prolonged discussion of problems and their history in favor of discussion potential solutions, MI promotes evocation of change talk and avoidance of sustain talk. Thus, there may be some overlapping mechanisms of change operating in these two models.

What differentiates the models is that MI practitioners may spend more time evoking change talk about motivation prior to transitioning to talking about next steps. In solution-focused therapy, this process may happen rapidly when the focus is on generating action steps, or solutions, that are already within the grasp of clients. Thus, MI will spend more time on the *why* of change and may be slower to get to the *how* of change than solution-focused therapy. Spending more time reviewing client's motivation for change can avoid a potentially detrimental focus on rushing to solve problems. Future researchers working with solution-focused therapy models may consider whether the timing of generating solutions impacts outcomes and whether adding MI in the engagement phase of solution-focused therapy may improve outcomes.

Because of their similarities, some have called for the integration of the two models (Lewis & Osborne, 2004), with some promising hybrid models showing effectiveness. Smith and Hall's (2008) strengths-oriented family therapy model (SOFT) blended MI, solution-focused therapy, and behavioral multifamily group work. SOFT was efficacious at reducing adolescent substance use through 6 months, and adherence to the model in the engagement phase predicted treatment entry (Smith et al., 2006, 2009).

Ecological Family Therapies

Family therapy researchers began translating the ecological framework of Urie Bronfrenbrenner in the 1980s and 1990s. What followed was a proliferation of hybrid family therapy models that included elements of structural and systemic interventions with a new focus on the ecology of the family. As Bronfrenbrenner's (1977) idea began as a model of human development, it is not surprising that many of these therapies focus on families with adolescents, including multidimensional family therapy (Liddle & Hogue, 2000), multisystemic family therapy (Henggeler & Schaeffer, 2019), and brief strategic family therapy (Szapocznik & Williams, 2000). Sprenkle (2012) noted that family intervention research was the most advanced with youth suffering from conduct or substance use disorders but critiqued the developers' ability to provide ecological family intervention trainings to most marriage and family therapy programs' graduate students.

Focus on extrafamilial intervention targets is no longer the unique domain of models that treat youth with externalizing problems. For example, the American Association for Marriage and Family Therapy (2004) includes case management among the professional competencies required for students trained in accredited programs. Although family workers cannot be all things to all people, we must recognize the external systems that affect our clients outside of our offices. Additionally, myriad new initiatives exist to coordinate care beyond traditional case management services at the structural level of health care, including wraparound services, integrated behavioral health services, and health homes.

Therapeutic Techniques

Regarding case management, at minimum helpers should know how to refer families to needed services and coordinate care with other professionals. In more intensive models, transportation may be provided to families, or helpers may accompany members to appointments (e.g., housing, unemployment office, hearing at a school board meeting). The box below describes one of my personal experiences advocating for families under the general rubric of case management activities.

Client Advocacy with School Administration

I collaborated with a 17-year-old client and their family. The youth had violated their school's substance use policy. Their highly distressed parents asked me to speak with the school administration on their behalf. The parents were concerned about expulsion and their child's ability to participate in prosocial activities at school. I agreed to accompany them to meet with school leadership.

The school administration worried that, if they allowed this student to remain involved in school activities despite the policy violation, they would then have to use this approach with all students. In response, I discussed the nature of addiction as a chronic-relapsing brain disorder for some individuals. I also argued that school policies that cut students off from prosocial activities, such as sports or clubs, could inadvertently result in increased substance use by students. That is, such students would now have less structured time with non-substance-using activities and more time to use substances. We now have more evidence that punitive school discipline predicts future teen substance use (Prins et al., 2023).

Ultimately, the school allowed the student to retain their privileges. Furthermore, by attending the school administration meeting, I believe this activity also enhanced my relationship with the family.

THOUGHT QUESTIONS: (1) What organizational policies affect your clients?
(2) Sometimes advocacy efforts are perceived as "enabling" a client or "working harder than a client." However, those who believe in providing case management view it as enhancing their clients' outcomes. What are your opinions/experiences regarding these conflicting ideas on the appropriateness of some case management activities?

Opportunities for Integration with MI

Client ambivalence is not the only mechanism operating in effective family work. At times, we should consider broadening the MI spirit to case management opportunities. Using case management strategies outside of the office conveys compassion and empathy. Prior definitions of compassion and empathy in the MI community only address helpers' verbal behavior in sessions, such as the use of affirmations or reflections that convey warmth and understanding of the family member. However, as case management acknowledges the broader systems that impact family members' lives, I argue for its inclusion in a broader conceptualization of empathy and compassion within the context of ecological family models.

Ambivalence is not the only mechanism operating in family work.

SUMMARY

This chapter reviewed key principles in family work and highlighted opportunities for integrating MI with various theoretical models. Despite differences in theoretical orientations, emphasis on process research is a common thread across these models. That is, most family therapy research has sought to determine what elements of family therapy results in outcomes. This jibes well with MI's process research on feedback loops between clinicians and clients within sessions, and how such interactions predict subsequent outcomes.

In Chapters 7 through 11, we will discuss application of MI's microcounseling skills to family work, as well as how to conceptualize change talk in this context. Then, we will turn our attention to integrating MI during various phases of family work, such as at the beginning, middle, and end of the helping relationship. I've organized these chapters around the four tasks of MI: engaging, focusing, engaging, and planning.

CHAPTER 7

Advanced Issues in Using ROARS with Families

> Those who would learn to fly one day must first learn to stand and walk and run and climb and dance. One cannot fly into flying.
> —Friedrich Nietzsche

When learning complex skills, most of us first learn general principles and then move to more complex applications. In Chapter 4, I presented the basic micro-counseling skills of MI with the acronym ROARS, which stands for reflections, open questions, affirmations, and reflective summaries. In this chapter, I address applications of these skills to a more complex situation, the family context.

There are some important differences between doing MI in family work and doing MI in individual sessions. In this chapter, we will talk about the need to **pivot** frequently among multiple individuals in the room, as well as define variations in MI micro-counseling skills that may be better suited for family sessions. I introduce the distinction between helper statements directed at individuals versus those directed at the broader family members. I call the latter **family-level ROARS** statements, and for the sake of simplicity will refer to the former just as ROARS.

PIVOT OFTEN

One key principle in using MI is to foster empathic relationships with all people we work with. Thus, a key consideration is whether doing individually focused MI with one family member during a session can risk disengagement or relational ruptures with another. From clinical experiences with both family and group work, I generally recommend refraining from doing individual work in front of other family members (Smith & Hall, 2010). There is too much potential for disengagement from other parties present if they are sitting idly while the helper singles out one person.

In using ROARS with families (or any groups, really), helpers need to dynamically rotate their attention among those present in the room. I call this *pivoting*. Making sure all parties are heard and engaged is necessary for creating an atmosphere of acceptance for the family unit as a whole. Extended evocation and praise directed toward one individual can raise another family members' ire, especially if there is acrimony between them.

Listening thoroughly to one individual, and creatively reflecting the content back, is hard enough. Yet, it is much easier than bouncing back and forth between multiple people sitting in your office. Pivoting takes energy and attention to track the views of multiple family members. The challenge of using MI in family work is understanding multiple perspectives and strategically responding to them all in real time. Learning how to quickly pivot between multiple parties will be essential if you are attempting to resolve the ambivalence of two or more people in your presence. Pivoting remains a foundational skill in both group (Wagner & Ingersoll, 2012) and family work (Smith & Hall, 2010).

Using MI in family work means understanding and responding to multiple perspectives at the same time.

Pivoting should feel dynamic. As opposed to conducting a one-on-one session with an audience, we aim to have an ongoing conversation with multiple people simultaneously. That may mean that, in some instances, a helper will, in a single breath, affirm one family member and then rapidly turn attention to another family member with another component of ROARS. An example of a helper using ROARS with individuals in quick succession, pivoting rapidly, would look like the following: "You are putting so much effort into communication and are starting to see some real payoffs at home," to one family member, allowing them to briefly respond, and then immediately pivoting to another family member with the open question "And how have things been for you since our last session?" A chief task of conjoint family work is rotating between family members while maintaining a coherent focus within the session.

Another useful way of efficiently speaking to the whole family, without necessarily pivoting, would be aiming statements at the family as a whole. Again, I define these helper behaviors as family-level ROARS skills.

FAMILY-LEVEL ROARS

Reflections, open questions, affirmations, and reflective summaries, or ROARS can all be adapted to speak to multiple members simultaneously. One of the key distinctions between individual- and family-level ROARS is that the latter include words such as "both of you" or "as a family" to cue the family members to your addressing them as a group.

Family-Level Affirmations

An example of a family-level affirmation could be "*You both* really are doing your best. That's admirable." Notice how, rather than simply affirming one party in the presence of the other, you are addressing both parties. If more than two people are present, you can simply adapt the stem of the affirmation to "*You are all . . .*" With affirmations, be especially mindful of situations where intense conflict exists between family members. In that situation, individual-level affirmations may backfire, and family-level affirmations may be preferable. In the next chapter, we will demonstrate how using individual affirmations can backfire using a family mediation example.

Family-Level Reflections

Similarly, family-level reflections address more than one individual at a time. An example could be "So, *all of you* share a common goal of improving communication and see a lot of benefits in making improvements there." Note how this reflection possesses potential for evoking change talk, as the helper ended the statement on the idea that the family would benefit from a change not yet made. By letting this hang in the air, it is hoped that this type of statement will prompt discussion of such benefits, which can then be reinforced and further elaborated.

One situation we should anticipate when using family-level reflections is that one family member may respond with change talk, and another may respond with sustain talk. At times, we can be working with both individual-level and family-level ambivalence. This necessitates pivoting. When one person responds, the helper can simply reply to that individual and then pivot while staying with the same theme. Consider the following example of using a *family-level ROARS* statement and then pivoting among family members.

Helper: So, all of you share a common goal of improving communication and see tangible benefits of becoming a better-oiled machine. [Complex reflection, reinforcing change talk]

Mom: Well, I'm less enthusiastic than the others, but I'm willing to give it a go. [Sustain talk]

Helper: So, you're lukewarm. This is hard for you. It's not natural for you to come see someone like me and it scares you. It's getting real now that we're talking about specific changes the family may ask you to make. Yet, you came here. [Double-sided reflection] And how do the rest of you feel about Mom trying? [Family-level open question]

Child: I think she feels the most stress about this and has already tried so much, that she's tired.

Helper: So, you acknowledge how hard your mom is working and appreciate her being here. [Complex reflection] Would you please do me a favor and say that directly to her? She may like to hear that directly from you.

Child: (*to the mom*) I'm also scared of where this is going but glad you came.

Helper: (*to the mom*) How was that for you? [Open question]

Mom: (*Tearfully shrugs and smiles.*)

Helper: (*to the dad*) And what do you make of your spouse's willingness to give this a shot?

Dad: I think her coming says a lot. She is tired, but we're here with her. I feel like just saying this out loud together is making us closer.

> One family member may respond with change talk and another with sustain talk.

Helpers make choices on the direction of the session every time they respond to a client statement. Here, the helper chose to integrate every family member in the discussion of one family member's ambivalence about a stated family goal, working on family communication. This is in direct contrast to having more of a one-on-one interaction with the parent in front of their spouse and child, exploring their ambivalence. Pivoting to other family members here had the added benefit of the ambivalent parent hearing their child and spouse's appreciation for them, which may further their motivation toward working on the goal.

In addition to using double-sided reflections to address one individual, as done in the example, they can also be adapted to reflect the content of multiple family members simultaneously. This is essentially a strategy for pivoting. As you recall, helpers use double-sided reflections with individuals to present back both sides of their ambivalence. In the example above, we noted how the parent was having a hard time with family work and also noted that, despite such difficulties or unnaturalness, they were sticking to it. A double-sided reflection highlighted both sides of the individual's ambivalence. In individual MI, these are useful for adroitly moving the conversation away from sustain talk toward change talk, as was the helper's goal above. In this example, the helper reflects the sustain talk (i.e., difficulty with accepting the family communication work goal) in the first portion of the statement, and their change talk (i.e., perseverance in the face of this hesitation) in the second.

By contrast, **family-level double sided reflections** first comment on one family member, and then rapidly pivot to another. Grammatically, think of this as a comma-separated clause wherein the first clause you address one person and after the comma you address a second person (e.g., You . . . , and you . . .). An example appears in Table 7.1: "You desperately need time to unwind, and you (other spouse) feel that you want them to be more present." This rapidly communicates that you are listening to both parties, without extensive, and potentially alienating, focus on just one person.

In individual sessions, double-sided reflections juxtapose sustain and change talk. In family-level double-sided reflections, the perspectives of different people comprise the two "sides." This particular reflection highlights the different perspectives of family members, not ambivalence. It is not necessarily getting at change talk yet, but it is conveying empathy to two individuals in conflict simultaneously. In the example above, this type of reflection is also pointing out competing needs in conflict, which, by definition, represents systemic thinking about a problem.

> In family-level double-sided reflections, the perspectives of different people comprise the two "sides."

In short, family-level reflections are statements helpers use to convey empathy or evoke change talk from multiple family members at one time. Excepting the double-sided subtype, family-level reflections share common stems signifying they are aimed at the family unit. Examples of these stems include "Both of you . . . ," "As a couple . . . ," or "As a family . . . ." Exercise 7.1 (end of chapter) is for practicing family-level reflections.

Family-Level Open Questions

Open questions that address multiple parties, and are not specifically directed at an individual, I call *family-level open questions*. Open questions are individually focused if they are specifically directed at one individual. Sometimes, helpers cue a specific person to answer by saying their

TABLE 7.1. Maintaining Family-Level Equipoise with Family-Level ROARS

Scenario: A married couple, Beth and Deborah, are working on their communication. The conversation lands on how social media use and computer gaming interferes with the quality of the time they spend together.

Purpose: Notice how individually focused reflections addressed to Beth can negatively affect Deborah. Observe the difference when the helper responds with family-level reflections. Family level reflections can be used to maintain family-level equipoise.

Individually focused reflections

Beth's statement	Helper reflection	Deborah's reaction
"What does it matter if I'm on my phone after dinner? It's how I unwind."	"You need time to unwind and are doing it the best way you know how."	Deborah may feel anger that the focus is on Beth's need to "unwind."
"I'm willing to cut down on gaming, but when Deborah nags me, it makes me just want to game more."	"You'd like there to be less nagging. You don't like that. And you're willing to cut down on gaming to make that happen."	Although the emphasis is on Beth's change talk here, it still may convey some blame on Deborah for "nagging."
"But if I put down the game, all they want to do is watch TV and not talk. I'm an extrovert living with an introvert, and the game is part of my coping."	"For you, the current alternative isn't much better."	Feeling blamed for Beth's gaming.

Family-level reflections

Beth's statement	Helper reflection	Deborah's reaction
"What does it matter if I'm on my phone after dinner? It's how I unwind."	"You desperately need time to unwind (*to Beth*), and you (*to Deborah*) feel that you want them to be more present."	The helper is responding to both Beth and Deborah, guessing at how this affects Deborah.
"I'm willing to cut down on gaming, but when Deborah nags me, it makes me just want to game more."	"You both aren't getting what you want and are both suffering from that."	Deborah's feelings are also acknowledged. She suffers, too!
"But if I put down the game, all they want to do is watch TV and not talk. I'm an extrovert living with an introvert and the game is part of my coping."	"You both have different needs, which are both valid. You both want to figure out how to get unstuck from this pattern."	Both Beth's and Deborah's needs are labeled as "valid." The second reflection also invites Deborah into a conversation about change.

name or by looking at them directly, which also prompts an individual to respond. An example of a *family-level open question* could be if a helper said, "So, what are some of your ideas, as a family, on how you may want to move forward?" You may recall that this particular question maps nicely onto the MI Spirit dimension of partnership, which involves inviting family member input into designing the agenda for sessions, deciding on the best route to change, and other forms of power sharing in the context of the helper–client relationship.

Family-Level Reflective Summaries

A distinguishing feature of a family-level reflective summary is that it will touch on the actions or statements of multiple family members. However, they may contain a blend of statements that address the family as a whole and specific individuals. For illustration purposes, let us continue the previous example earlier in the chapter of a family working on improving their communications.

HELPER: So, today, *you all* did a lot, and it seems like *you're all* starting to get a clearer picture of where you want to go as a family and some specific things you want out of our time together. [Family-level statement] One of the highlights for me was the remarkable exchange when we started clarifying the goal of working on family communication. I heard you (*to the mom*) openly talk about some hesitations about working on family communication, which I think is a great sign that she's taking some real risks. That's hard to say in front of your family and me. Staying silent about your true feelings would be an easy way out. Truly courageous. You two (*looking at other family members*) supported them by saying really nice things and further expressed your willingness to do some work and stand side-by-side with them in a scary adventure. That shows some great effort at showing affection. I'm not sure how you all experienced it, but it was heartwarming for me to watch, as you all seemed to bond over this exchange today. What are your thoughts for how to build upon today's work?

As mentioned above in the definition, this family-level summary is such because it comments on the actions and statements of multiple family members. Note that affirmations were simultaneously directed to the family unit, an individual, and a dyad within the larger family (i.e., second parent and child). Thus, it contains a mix of family-level ROARS and individually focused ROARS.

A family-level reflective summary incorporates actions and statements of multiple family members.

USING FAMILY-LEVEL ROARS TO ENGAGE AND ADDRESS AMBIVALENCE

If you are new to working with multiple people simultaneously, it may take some time to master family-level ROARS skills. Pivoting between people requires being able to track the perspectives of multiple people, and then form coherent replies. This is no small task.

As you recall, MI is used to address and resolve ambivalence toward behavior change in a warm, nonconfrontational manner. In Exercise 7.1, I provide a practice activity that is designed to help with both identifying change talk and identifying family-level ROARS skills.

SUMMARY

In individually focused MI, the micro-counseling skills, or ROARS, are all addressed directly to an individual. Here, we discussed adaptations of these skills for use in pivoting among family members in situations where multiple people are present in the helping room. Pivoting was presented as a critical skill that could be used to enhance motivation, engage all parties, and prevent any ill feelings that may arise from taking more of an individual focus in front of a family audience. Overreliance on talking to one family member may risk alienating another. Simply put, if you do individual therapy in front of accompanying family members, you may show empathy only for that individual. By using family-level ROARS, you can convey empathy to multiple people simultaneously.

Sometimes, using family-level ROARS is as simple as addressing reflections and questions to multiple parties by adding qualifying wording such as "both of you," or "as a family," or "as a couple."

The next chapter addresses how we can conceptualize and address change talk in the family context. I present some complexities in dealing with varying levels of ambivalence across family members.

EXERCISE 7.1. Making Family-Level MI Responses

Instructions: Imagine a parent and teenage child who are in constant conflict. You are a child protection worker who is providing preventative services to the family. The child and the parent are also attending individually focused services that address anger management skills and parenting skills, respectively. You meet with them conjointly to track their progress. In this exercise, read the client statement on the left, and attempt to write a reflection or affirmation at the family rather than individual level. To help you, I have inserted some suggested stems you may consider using, but don't feel confined to them if you have other ways of wording responses.

Client statement	Helper statement
1. Child: "I feel like I can't breathe when my mom asks me five times to do something."	1. "You feel _____, and your mom feels _____."
2. Mom: "She lost her temper and punched a hole in the wall. That's when I knew we needed help. And she'll admit it, too, that things got out of hand."	2. "You feel _____, and you both _____"
3. Child: "Yeah, but I wouldn't do that shit if my mom wasn't such a jerk sometimes. I mean, I'm doing my part in those anger classes."	3. "You're _____, and you're hoping that you both _____."
4. Mom: "I have seen her make some small changes. Not nearly enough, but small. I'm trying, too."	4. "You're both willing to _____."
5. Child: "If it means I can stop meeting with you and stop going to those dumb classes, yes."	5. "You want _____," and I bet you (*to Mom*) want _____."
6. Mom: "Well, I think we need to stick with all this until things change. But yes, it's a big hassle."	6. "You both _____."
7. Child: "You never give me enough credit for how much I'm doing. I'm trying, but it's never enough."	7. "So, to recap, you (*to child*) _____," and you (*to Mom*) _____. So, what do each of you want to try next?"

CHAPTER 8

Change Talk among Families

> If the family were a boat, it would be a canoe
> that makes no progress unless everyone paddles.
> —Letty Cottin Pogrebin

In the prior chapter, I addressed some complexities of using ROARS skills in the family context. Here, I cover the more specific task of listening for and reinforcing language in the direction of change, or change talk, when multiple parties are present in the room.

In individually focused MI, helpers usually address a single target behavior. So, this raises some key questions when adapting this process to family members. Does change talk exist at both the individual and family levels? Can using evocative strategies result in strong bonds with some family members, but weaken bonds with other family members? Are multiple individual target behaviors all present and requiring selective reinforcement in the dance that is family work? In my view, the answer to these questions is a resounding YES!

Here, I present a conceptualization of how both individual and **family-level change talk** may be addressed in family work. Note that my articulation here is largely theoretical in nature because little work exists in this area. Thus, it is my hope that it will be a launching pad for empirical and clinical work by those interested in using MI with families.

Let's start this chapter by revisiting the concept of equipoise, defined earlier as remaining neutral with regards to identifying and reinforcing family member change talk. Please recall that we use equipoise in situations where it may be unethical to pursue change talk. To illustrate the concept of equipoise I use an example drawn from family mediation work. Then, I discuss what we currently know about change talk from research on family therapy. Finally, I present a conceptual model for addressing change talk in family work.

EQUIPOISE IN FAMILY WORK

Chapter 5 discussed the central role of evoking change talk in resolving client ambivalence. That is, the helper's role in MI involves eliciting change talk, or client speech pertaining to change (e.g., "I want to be here, so my daughter and I aren't always fighting") when there is ambivalence about a particular course of action. Once elicited it is reinforced, spotlighting family members' motivations toward change. So, in essence, MI is directive in that we attempt to nudge family members in specific directions, toward some change that is beneficial to them. Yet, nudging toward change should be constrained within the boundaries of our compassion. For some ambivalence-addled decisions, helpers should refrain from generating and reinforcing change talk for ethical reasons. In these situations, helpers can still abide by the MI Spirit and make masterful use of the ROARS microcounseling skills. However, because they are not pursuing change talk, we refer to this as maintaining *equipoise* within MI (Miller & Rollnick, 2012).

Miller and Rollnick (2012) introduced the concepts of *equipoise* and *compassion* in the third edition of the seminal text on MI. This came after years of hard lessons about the potential for using MI to sway people to make certain decisions. As you recall, compassion refers to keeping the clients' interests central. For example, it would likely be unethical to systematically elicit and reinforce change talk in the direction of making a decision about divorce (e.g., "So, it sounds like your life would be better if you ended things"). As helpers, it is impossible to know whether marital dissolution would serve our clients best, whatever our professional judgment and individual biases. Privileging change talk in the direction of divorce would also conflict with the American Association for Marriage and Family Therapy's (2015) *Code of Ethics*, which states that clients should autonomously decide such matters. Regardless of whether helpers use other strategies in MI designed to boost autonomy (i.e., asking permission to give advice, telling clients they get to choose what to decide), equipoise is the preferred helper stance when seeing couples considering divorce.

Family-Level Equipoise

I define **family-level equipoise** as equal application of the MI Spirit and attention to change language across multiple people. Thus, this definition does not encompass the decision of whether change talk is strategically generated (Miller & Rollnick, 2023). To achieve family-level equipoise, one will have to pivot often and master family-level ROARS.

There are good reasons to achieve family-level equipoise. It prevents distressed family members from becoming disengaged. No family member should sit idly while they observe a long exchange between the helper and another. Additionally, sometimes excessive reinforcement on one member's change language will be off-putting to another family member, especially if they see the helper as siding with that individual versus them. Finally, when multiple family members are offering change language around a shared target behavior, pivoting adds depth to the conversation.

Family-level equipoise requires pivoting often.

Family Mediation Example

Family mediation represents an area of practice where equipoise is highly preferred. Family mediation occurs when divorcing couples attempt to avoid litigation over parenting and custody arrangements (Morris et al., 2018). Mediators work with both members of the couple, requiring a tightrope walk between maintaining neutrality and fostering mutually agreeable decisions. When couples are distributing property and/or making custody arrangements, significant hostility often exists between the parties. This could range from mildly confrontational "tit-for-tat" negotiating to a deep-seated reluctance to budge on anything that appears to favor the estranged partner.

Although MI holds much promise for use in family mediation, few concrete demonstrations exist (Blakely et al., 2017). So, let us contrast two different interactions. In this case, John and Maribeth are divorcing. They entered mediation to facilitate agreements about visitation times for their children, who are 10 and 12. Both parties felt spited by the other. They both claimed that the other parent deliberately brought the children late to their visits, depriving them of precious time. Additionally, they each claimed that the other parent used them as an "on-call babysitter" when it suited them, so they could have more free time at the other's expense.

For illustrative purposes, I present two versions of a conversation with a couple. In the first example, a mediator uses strategies that violates the principle of *family-level equipoise*. Again, helper behaviors violate family-level equipoise when unequal attention is given to the MI Spirit and change talk for a single family member. See if you can identify where that happens during this brief exchange.

Example 1: Lack of Family-Level Equipoise

HELPER: So, tell me a little bit about what you're hoping to gain from meeting today. [Collaborative open question]

MARIBETH: We came here because *he* is doing petty things around visit times, and I'm now sinking to his level.

JOHN: Well, I'm glad you're at least calling both the pot and the kettle black.

HELPER: I'm hoping we can refrain from slinging mud at each other while we're here, and that goes both ways *(looking at Maribeth)*. We'll get to you soon, John. Right now, I'd like to hear Maribeth's perspective. Maribeth, you seem angry about what is happening and are also ready to take some responsibility because you want what is best for your kids. [Complex reflection] So, here we sit. That's admirable. [Affirmation] I'm sure it's not easy. Tell me why you want to use mediation to solve this. [Open question; evokes change talk]

MARIBETH: I suppose because we have to do something about bringing the kids to each other late. It's making us yell at each other, and our kids are old enough to know what's going on. It hurts them to see that. [Change talk—reason]

HELPER: So, although it is hard to be in a room with John, you're willing to work something out to spare your kids some real pain. Enough is enough. [Complex reflection]

MARIBETH: Yes. After arguments, we see the kids withdraw and spend hours on their phones and not talk to us, which sets a foul mood for the short time each of us has to spend with them.

HELPER: So, reducing arguments on handoffs may make your time with the kids get better, which would be good for you. [Complex reflection]

MARIBETH: I think so. And I just can't live with all this anger. I'm not an angry person.

HELPER: You don't like how expressing anger to John makes you feel about yourself. It's not how you envision yourself. [Complex reflection]

MARIBETH: Yes, but I just feel so out of control when we are doing handoffs.

HELPER: And you're the type of person who wants to take things in stride. That's a great trait. [Affirmation]

MARIBETH: Yeah *(smiling and sighing)*.

HELPER: So, you have many reasons to think about what you personally can do on your side to avoid arguments. [Simple reflection, reinforcing change talk]

MARIBETH: Yes, I almost wonder if we should ask our parents to do the dropoffs, so we avoid seeing each other. Then, if they're late, we're not at each other's throats. [Change talk—activation]

HELPER: That's really a great idea, Maribeth. [Affirmation] You're willing to problem solve this and do whatever it takes to protect those kids from seeing you two get angry at each other. [Reflection, reinforcing change talk] That's really admirable of you that you're seeing past your feelings for the greater good . . . for the kids. [Affirmation] And John, you've been sitting quietly. What do you think about all this? [Open question]

JOHN: Well, first off, I'm only getting into arguments that she starts. And she was a *way* angry person during our whole marriage. That's bullshit that her anger is just situational. You make it sound like she's all protecting the kids and got their best interest at heart, but she's manipulating them against me. No offense, but I think family therapists, judges, and lawyers all just side with mothers.

The helper did wonderful MI, but only with Maribeth. Here, the target behavior is "not being late when dropping children off to a former spouse." Although the target behavior applies to two people, only one received significant focus in this short excerpt. Figure 8.1 shows a schematic of how there is a lack of pivoting.

The helper drew out Maribeth's change talk by using reflections and open questions and poured on affirmations and reflections to reinforce it. For example, the helper elicited some of Maribeth's reasons for wanting to solve this problem (e.g., "Tell me why you want to use mediation . . . "). The helper also reinforces Maribeth's potential solution of asking parents for help by saying it was a good idea. So, this is clearly MI centered on change talk at the individual level, and not equipoise.

This dialogue, however, violates the principle of family-level equipoise defined earlier in the chapter. By giving unequal attention to the MI Spirit and change talk across parties, John was left out too long. This short exchange with Maribeth enraged him. Why is that? One possibility is that positively affirming Maribeth in front of John came at the expense of alienating him. You see this when he makes a clear statement that everyone is against him and not seeing his perspective. So, even though the helper provided competent individually

One family member's affirmation should never be another family member's confrontation.

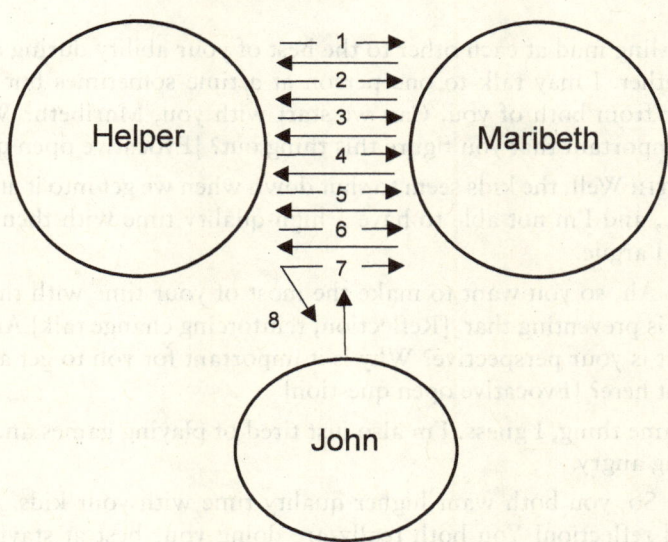

FIGURE 8.1. No pivoting: Individually focused MI while a family member waits/observes.

focused MI with Maribeth, it was akin to doing individual therapy in front of a bystander. Empathically eliciting change talk from one member can, at times, lower partnership with another family member. One family member's affirmation should never be another family member's confrontation.

This exchange would put the helper in the unenviable position of having to backtrack and establish empathy with John. Maintaining family-level equipoise helps avoid this thorny issue. So, what would family-level equipoise look like for this case?

Example 2: Preserving Family-Level Equipoise in Family Mediation

HELPER: I'm so glad you both came in today. From what you said on the phone, you want to come to an agreement about some problems with dropoff times for your kids. You both really want to avoid having to take each other to court. [Reinforcing prior session change talk] So, I hope we can talk through this. Given the problems you mentioned on the phone, I can imagine this being hard for both of you to be here but want to give you a shout out for doing something difficult for the sake of your kids. That shows a lot of character for both of you. [Family-level affirmation] So, I'd like to start by asking both of you to please not sling mud at each other to the best of your ability during our time together. I may talk to one person at a time sometimes but want to hear from both of you. Can we start with you, Maribeth? Why is it so important that you figure this thing out? [Evocative open question]

MARIBETH: Well, the kids seem to shut down when we get into it at dropoff time, and I'm not able to have a high-quality time with them if John and I argue.

HELPER: Ah, so you want to make the most of your time with them, and this is preventing that. [Reflection, reinforcing change talk] And John, what is your perspective? Why is it important for you to get an agreement here? [Evocative open question]

JOHN: Same thing, I guess. I'm also just tired of playing games and always being angry.

HELPER: So, you both want higher-quality time with your kids. [Family-level reflection] You both really are doing your best at staying close to them during this difficult situation. That's admirable. [Family-level affirmation] And John, there is something more to it, too. How would things get better for you if you weren't always angry? [Open question, evoking change talk]

JOHN: I'd feel more relaxed, I guess.

HELPER: That's great. And I'm wondering if you think you'd feel more relaxed, too, Maribeth, if we get some agreements in place about this? [Closed question]

MARIBETH: I think so. I mean, this was a messy divorce. I still sometimes just feel something in the pit of my stomach whenever I see John.

JOHN: No kidding.

HELPER: If you decide to solve this (*addressing both Maribeth and John*), you both may also need to figure out a strategy that works for you to manage visitations. That plan may be different for each of you, and really, we're here to talk about agreements, but you both may possibly be interested in pursuing this outside of mediation. [Complex reflection]

MARIBETH AND JOHN: (*Nod.*)

HELPER: So, if that is something that interests you, I have some suggestions that I'm happy to share with each of you privately. [Autonomy respect] I'm really impressed with how well you two are doing right now managing those gut feelings. I think it shows you are both committed to talking about how we may handle your dropoff problems and shows a lot of strength. It is easier to do what you always do and get mad, but you're putting that aside right now because you don't want to always feel so angry and want more quality time with your kids. [Affirmation-reinforcing commitment] So, what are some of your ideas on how you may want to handle dropoffs differently? [Open question, eliciting activation and taking steps]

The first dialogue example showed when it is inappropriate to have an imbalance in affirming and also eliciting and reinforcing change talk in a conjoint session. The second example demonstrates dynamic pivoting. Figure 8.2 illustrates the pivoting between John and Maribeth.

The example focuses on a situation where two people are in the room. This raises the question of which situations call for eliciting individual change talk in family work. Clearly, parties seeking family mediation are at odds with each other. Yet, in some scenarios, it may be more appropriate to generate and reinforce change language from an individual, even when others in the family are present. For example, consider the partner reluctant to attend family sessions or a family member who is ambivalent about making changes requested by others. In these scenarios, the change talk of the reluctant family member would likely be music to the other

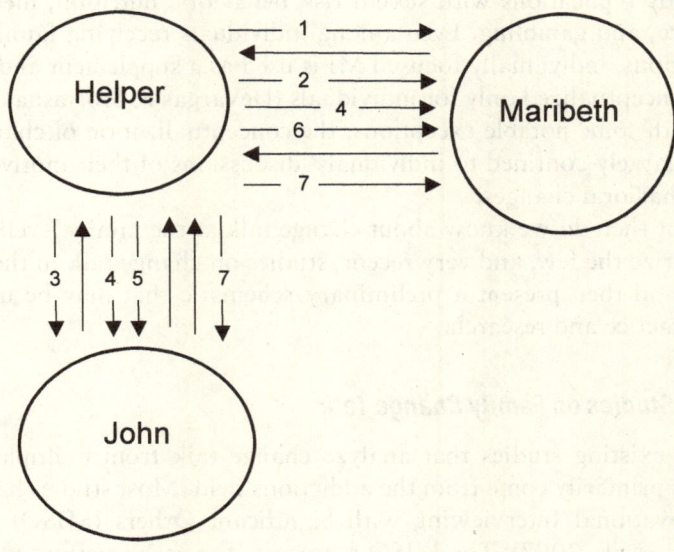

FIGURE 8.2. Dynamic pivoting to each family member in attendance.

family members' ears. Additionally, meeting one on one with family members may be the best course of action sometimes. Here, the helper would still be working systemically toward the end of greater family member participation. Getting more family members to participate could benefit the **identified client** and the entire family (Sprenkle et al., 2009). As you recall, I define the identified client as the person that either presents to treatment first or has the diagnosable condition that prompted services.

In other situations where entire families are working together, eliciting change talk at the family level may be appropriate. To some extent, whether a helper decides to work with an individual who is being scapegoated by the rest of the family, or start with everyone in the room, depends on how much family conflict exists. I address various patterns of family engagement in Chapter 9.

CHANGE TALK IN FAMILY WORK

Currently, change talk is almost always conceptualized at the individual level. Research shows that, when individuals have proportionally higher change talk than sustain talk, they are more likely to make changes for the target behavior in question (Magill et al., 2018). Although the majority of studies on change talk predict future alcohol or drug use from it, there exist study replications with sexual risk behaviors, nutrition, medication adherence, and gambling. Even among individuals receiving family-based interventions, individually focused MI is used as a supplement and change talk is conceptualized only for individuals (DeVargas & Stormshak, 2020). Thus, with some notable exceptions, the conceptualization of change talk remains largely confined to individuals' discussions of their motivation to make behavioral changes.

What then do we know about change talk at the family level? Below, I summarize the few, and very recent, studies on change talk in the family context and then present a preliminary schematic that may be useful in future practice and research.

Existing Studies on Family Change Talk

The few existing studies that analyze change talk from multiple family members primarily come from the addictions field. Most studies have used the Motivational Interviewing with Significant Others (MISO) manual (Apodaca et al., 2007). The MISO represents the earliest effort to date to adapt individually focused MI process measures for use with families.

Fokas et al. (2020) analyzed couples' change talk during behavioral couples therapy for alcoholism in both the first session and in the middle of treatment (i.e., Session 8 or 9). Surprisingly, significant other change talk early in session one predicted higher identified patient sustain talk later in that same session. These authors interpreted this finding as meaning that the identified patient, the one with the alcohol problem, possibly recoiled from their partner's change language, hearing it as pressure to change. In turn, they responded with sustain language, reflecting their state of ambivalence about changing their alcohol use. This is consistent with my concept of family-level equipoise, where attention to one person's change talk may negatively influence other family members in the room. This may be especially true in early sessions, per this study.

However, in this study, things changed during later sessions. At mid-treatment, significant other change talk predicted subsequent identified patient change talk within the same session. Decreases in mid-treatment sustain language from the identified patient was associated with more days of abstinence. Significant other change language, however, did not predict identified patient drinking at follow up. It is also notable that the authors discussed the difficulty in coding significant other sustain language, so it was omitted from analyses in this study. What is remarkable about this study is that it requires us to think about how eliciting change talk for one person in the family system may sometimes be detrimental to other family members.

Fokas et al. (2020) analyzed change talk in the context of a bona fide couples therapy model. Other studies analyzed the contribution of significant other change and sustain language in the context of a brief intervention that mainly targets the identified patient. These brief interventions lasted far fewer sessions (i.e., one to four sessions) and did not explicitly seek to do family therapy per se. Rather, they invited one's romantic partner to join as an adjunct to the otherwise individually focused session(s). For example, in Project MATCH, one of the largest studies of alcoholism treatment to date, adults receiving motivational enhancement therapy (MET) could optionally bring a significant other to one of their four MI sessions. Only 34.7% of participants had a significant other attend at least one session. In one small analysis of audio recordings from Project MATCH's MET sessions ($n = 27$; 81.5% romantic partners), significant other sustain talk, but not change talk, predicted identified patient drinking intensity (Manuel et al., 2012). An additional secondary analysis of Project MATCH data extended these findings by using longer follow-up time. Similar to the other studies, significant other change talk did not predict identified patient drinking, but their sustain language did (Bourke et al., 2016). Finally, Apodaca et al. (2013) analyzed how statements by concerned significant others (CSOs, consisting of 41% romantic partners, 30% friends, and 29% family members) in favor of or against the identified patient reducing alcohol use impacted their change talk. Identified patient change talk was more likely following CSO statements in favor of change. Notably, these authors called the CSO statements "support change" or "against change," referring only to the identified patient's single target behavior of reducing alcohol use.

In fact, all these recent studies presume one target behavior that resides in one individual, even though family members are in the room ostensibly engaging in change talk or supporting another's change. This shows the current ambivalence among clinicians about how to conceptualize change talk at the dyadic or family level. As described here and in Chapter 5, change talk always occurs in the context of a target behavior. So, if an individual is ambivalent about making changes in their drug use, change talk would refer to any pro-change client language, such as "I'm going to delete my dealer's number in my phone." Currently, family member change talk is anything that supports this individual in making this individual change (e.g., "Yes, I'm proud of them for cutting ties to substance users. I know it's hard."). Thus, family member change talk currently has been conceptualized only as supporting the identified client's goal. Starks et al. (2018) call this an "identified-client" framework, as family members are present but mainly focused on one individual's target behavior.

Conceptualizing change talk as an individual matter conflicts with family systems thinking. Doing so essentially ignores any family dynamics besides those that directly interface with one member's target behavior. In individually focused MI, there is no effort to frame the target behavior systemically for the family, a cornerstone in much family work (Nichols & Davis, 2020). Thus, new models are needed that expand beyond this identified-client framework of change talk.

Family-Level Change Talk

Multiple Target Behaviors Are Normal

Just as I described the need to pivot frequently between various family members, helpers should be prepared to pivot between target behaviors in family work. Multiple target behaviors can be addressed in conjoint family sessions, or helpers may elect to focus on one single target behavior per session.

In this conceptualization, the timing of switching between target behaviors becomes an important consideration, as MI relies on a degree of processing depth to build motivation for each behavior. It is not yet established if it is better to build in-depth motivation for a single behavior, or if it is okay to develop a modicum of change language across multiple targets if they all lead to big picture change, because most process studies focus on single target behavior implementations of MI.

Notwithstanding the complexities of doing MI with families, switching between target behaviors in family work may feel liberating for many of us who have been reluctant to explore topics previously considered ancillary that come up in single target behavior examples of MI.

Defining Target Behaviors

Here, I define a **family-level target behavior** (FTB) as a family-level change that requires behavior changes from multiple family members. For example, consider a family that brings their child late to school every day. The FTB would be getting to school on time, and changes are needed from different family members (e.g., child going to bed earlier, parent arranging transportation, parent waking child up). These behaviors from individual family members could be conceptualized as **personal target behaviors** for each individual. However, if the personal target behavior is required by one member to achieve the FTB, I will call it a **multilevel target behavior** (MTB). I will reserve the term secondary personal target behavior for change decisions that mainly affect one individual and do not map neatly onto a family goal. Helpers can elicit and reinforce change talk in reference to the overall FTB or for MTBs. Again, following systems thinking, I assume there will be some degree of interdependence between family members' target behaviors.

FTB requires behavior changes from multiple family members.

Defining Change Talk in Family Work

When multiple people are attending conjoint family sessions, target behaviors—and, by corollary, change talk—may be best conceptualized as a series of statements varying in their level of interdependence. A **personal change talk** statement is one that seems more relevant for only one's own target behavior. I say "more relevant" because one of the key strategies in family work is to conceptualize problems systemically. So, arguably, no change talk statement is entirely bereft of the family context. An example of this may be working on ambivalence about engaging in grief therapy. So, imagine an individual pressured by their partner to work on grief, who was reluctant to come to therapy unless their partner attended with them.

Although a family member is present for support, this couple does not have any other family-level problems they are seeking to address in these sessions. Thus, change talk about doing certain things to overcome grief, such as ambivalence to even attend counseling, comes primarily from the grief-stricken partner, and anything the accompanying partner says is generally considered as change talk that maps onto that individual's problem. This is the current status quo in family-based change talk studies we reviewed earlier in this chapter.

Conversely, a **multilevel change talk** statement is one that maps onto both a personal target behavior and an FTB. You may already be asking what motivated the nongrieving partner in this example to seek out counseling. What if, in addition to grief, we add some relationship problems to the scenario? Let us now assume that the grief is exacerbating preexisting relationship problems such as communication and showing affection. The nongrieving partner senses emotional distance, and one intrapersonal issue is that this person thrives in relationships where affection is constantly shown. Because this is a systemic problem, it becomes the FTB. Thus, grief becomes a multilevel problem because it maps onto both personal target behavior and FTBs. So, here, change talk statements made about working on grief could be counted both in reference to grief outcomes as well as family functioning outcomes. For example, if the broader FTB is conceptualized as relationship enhancement, and the grieving partner says, "I'm willing to talk to someone about grief for the sake of our marriage," it would be considered change talk for two separate target behaviors. This is because it counts as a change talk statement for the personal goal of addressing grief, as well as a family-level change talk statement for the family goal of relationship enhancement. This is the essence of a multilevel change talk statement. In Figure 8.3, this "double-counted" change talk statement is represented by the overlapping region between personal and family levels. That region shows how target behaviors are multilevel, existing on two levels.

Personal change talk exists on a continuum in terms of how related it is to the FTB. When it is less related to the FTB, it sits in the rightmost region of Figure 8.3, where there is no overlap with the FTB. For example, a statement like "I want to work on my grief, so I'm less distracted at work" clearly counts as change talk toward the personal target behavior of working on grief, but it is yet unclear if it would predict whether the couple met their relationship enhancement goal. In the traditional change talk coding model, it likely would not count toward the FTB. However, the reason for referral is tied up in family pressure to get grief therapy, and grief therapy maps onto the FTB. So, a case could be made that the statement above

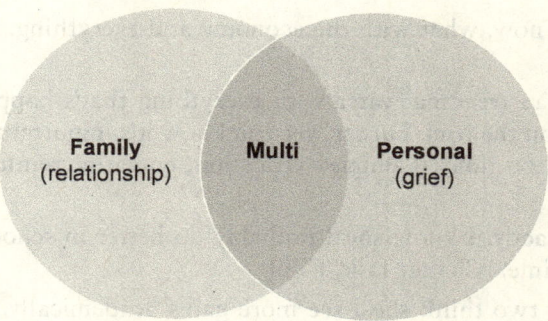

FIGURE 8.3. Overlap between family-level, multilevel, and personal target behaviors.

should predict the overall FTB. Future research should test whether this is the case.

To further delineate differences between personal and multilevel change talk statements in family work, let us examine a dialogue between two parents and a helper. This family was referred to a school social worker because of persistent tardiness to the first-period class at the beginning of the school day. The school social worker believes that the youth's tardiness is affecting other students, as they consider it one among many interruptions. Furthermore, the social worker believes that coming earlier would help the student settle down and focus better because they miss a mindfulness exercise at the beginning of the day. Thus, they feel that the student's grades may improve. I have annotated what I believe constitutes personal and multilevel change talk statements and also noted the target behaviors to which they are yoked.

HELPER: I want to thank you all for coming today and meeting with me. As you know, I wanted to talk about Diamond not making it to first period on time. [FTB] However, I also want to see if you have any other important topics you'd like to chat with me about while you're here. What else would be useful to your family? [Open question, enhancing partnership]

PARENT 1: I appreciate the way you say that. You know . . . part of the reason we can't get Diamond here on time is that I work overnights at the gas station. It's stressful. It's not that I don't want her to get there on time. [Change talk, FTB] It's just that I'm a hot mess. I cannot lose my job right now, what with the economy and everything. [Sustain talk, FTB]

HELPER: You're treading water with everything that's happening, and it gets put on the back burner, yet you know it's important for her to be at school on time. [Complex reflection, empathy, reinforcing change talk]

PARENT 1: Exactly. I know she'd probably do better in school if she were here on time. [Change talk, FTB]

HELPER: You two think she'd see more gains academically. [Family-level simple reflection, reinforcing change talk]

PARENT 2: Yeah, I do. [Change talk, FTB] But it's going to be impossible to always get her here on time. [Sustain talk, FTB] I cannot drive her either, and our bus takes 45 minutes from our neighborhood. She ain't ready early enough to catch it. I wish we could figure something out. [Change talk, FTB]

HELPER: So, I'm hearing from both of you that it is really important to you, and, despite the challenges, you're open to thinking more about how to make it happen. That's why you're here. [Family-level complex reflection]

PARENT 1: I think so. As long as any decision we come to is reasonable.

PARENT 2: Agreed.

PARENT 1: I also want a better job. [MTB] If I worked more normal hours, it would help me, and maybe I could get Diamond to school on time. [Change talk, FTB] And I'm sure you wouldn't mind either (*looking at Parent 2*).

PARENT 2: I'd get to see you so much more, and it would make our family life so much better.[1] I miss having more family time [Change talk, MTB], and it would be better for Diamond's schooling. [Change talk, FTB]

HELPER: So, one option that you've considered is switching work. It sounds like there may be some benefits to both Diamond getting here and also to you and your family. [Simple reflection, reinforcing change talk] If it's okay, let's focus on the Diamond aspect for a second. How would

---

[1] Since this change talk appears to relate to both the FTB (getting to school on time) and the parent's target behavior of getting a new job (MTB), it is highly interconnected. I think any change talk related to the MTB should also count toward the FTB, but more research is needed on this topic. For the sake of simplicity, I'm only annotating this as being change talk for the MTB.

Change Talk among Families

getting her to school on time benefit her? [Open question, evoking change talk]

PARENT 1: Honestly, I'm not sure it matters that much. I mean, what is the big deal being 10 minutes late each day. [Sustain talk, FTB] I think the new job mainly helps us all feel more connected and me feeling better. [Change talk, MTB]

HELPER: So, you're thrilled to do this, yet don't think it will really result in any gains at all if Diamond starts getting here earlier. [Complex reflection, amplification]

PARENT 2: I'm not sure I'd go that far. I think Diamond feels bad about being late. I actually feel like it makes her feel poor and ashamed. She knows she's not like better-off kids who get there on time. She knows we got to work late. [Change talk, FTB]

PARENT 1: And there's the school nagging us and leaving voicemails. That irritation would go away. [Change talk, FTB]

HELPER: For you two, you'd feel good to be left alone. One less hassle. [Family-level simple reflection] And you mentioned her possibly doing better academically if she arrived earlier. You want her to do well because she doesn't have some advantages other kids have. [Simple reflection, reinforcing change talk] Tell me how that would be for your family. [Evocative open question]

PARENT 2: We know she needs an education. Maybe if she felt good about doing well in school, she won't fall in with the wrong crowd later. You know we don't live in the best neighborhood. [Change talk, FTB]

HELPER: So, you want her to do better than kids typically do in your neighborhood, and maybe this is a small step that gives you hope about her future. [Complex reflection, reinforcing change talk] Now, let's turn back to how to get her here. You've mentioned one possible solution—you getting a new job that would allow you to get here on time and how that would improve your family life. Tell me more about how things would get better? [Evocative open question focused on MTB]

PARENT 1: I think if we were all on the same schedule, we could all eat dinner together. [Change talk, MTB]

PARENT 2: Yeah, we'd feel more like a family. Right now, it's just like we're roommates. [Change talk, MTB]

HELPER: Seems like that is a solution you really want to pursue. [Simple reflection, reinforcing change talk] So, on a scale of 1 to 10, with 10 being super confident and 1 being not so confident, how confident are you that you'll be able to get a new day job? [Scaling question, evoking change talk on MTB around ability]

PARENT 1: Maybe a 4.

HELPER: So, why a 4 and not a zero? [Open question, evoking change talk]

PARENT 1: I mean, when I look for a job, I don't leave any stone unturned. [Change talk, MTB]

Helper: When you make your mind up, you're hard working. It's one of your strengths. [Affirmation, reinforcing change talk]

PARENT 2: Yeah, she's hard-headed (*playfully joking*).

PARENT 1: Watch it (*smiling*).

HELPER: You guys are sweet. So, you do have some confidence that this may work. And you're starting to think that this direction will be good for both of you and for Diamond. [Complex reflection, reinforcing change talk for both MTB and FTB]

PARENT 1: Yeah, I agree. She'd get to school, and I'd get some normalcy back. [Change talk, MTB and FTB] She'd probably eat healthier in the morning, too, which may be good for her. At the gas station, she just gets junk food before school. [Change talk, MTB]

This example exposes the complexity of conceptualizing interdependent change talk statements for a behavior change that involves more than one person. Take, for example, the last statement made by Parent 1: "At the gas station, she just gets junk food before school." In current conceptualizations of change talk, it is actually unclear if this client statement would be considered change talk if we rigidly only considered getting her to school as the target behavior. That is because the statement is more in reference to what I call an MTB, getting a new job. However, it is possible that this statement indirectly counts as change talk toward the FTB (i.e., school tardiness) because of the interdependence between this and the mom's emerging goal of getting a new job. In other words, getting a job was offered as a potential solution to the FTB of school tardiness, which counts as change talk in reference to that goal. Yet, change talk then also emerged surrounding that particular goal. These interdependencies bring up challenges for how to conceptualize change talk in the family work context.

Note, too, that getting Diamond to school on time, the FTB, also requires some action on Diamond's part. It is yoked to Diamond, but she isn't even in the room! We did not address Diamond's motivation by eliciting her personal change talk. However, that could either be done in a family or individual session with Diamond present.

Note that, despite the complexities involved, the primary reason the school social worker contacted these parents was to discuss tardiness. So, that tardiness was the focus of most of the conversation. It is their specific charge as a school employee. It may be that the social worker may not continue working deliberately on the goals of job seeking or family togetherness due to time constraints or a lack of specific knowledge about bona fide family therapy. Yet, think about the potential ripple effect that this brief encounter could possibly have had on this family.

Finally, one possibility is that a family member indicates a personal goal that is twice removed from the FTB. I call this a **secondary personal target behavior**. For example, what if the parent in this example who wants a new job said that one benefit of this may be getting in shape? In other words, the new job (i.e., MTB) would not only allow them to spend more time with the family and get Diamond to school, but also help them get into shape. I think getting into shape would be counted as change talk toward the MTB of getting a job and the FTB. Getting in shape is a secondary personal target behavior that has little to do with the FTB. Thus, change talk from the parent about getting in shape would not be counted toward the FTB. As getting in shape only applies to one parent, extensive focus on change talk about that personal behavior (i.e., "How would you benefit from getting in shape?") in front of other family members may start to distract from the FTB. It could inhibit pivoting. Follow-up discussions about secondary personal target behaviors may be helpful when possible. Figure 8.4 shows how this type of secondary personal target behavior may be best saved for an individual session if a family goal takes center stage.

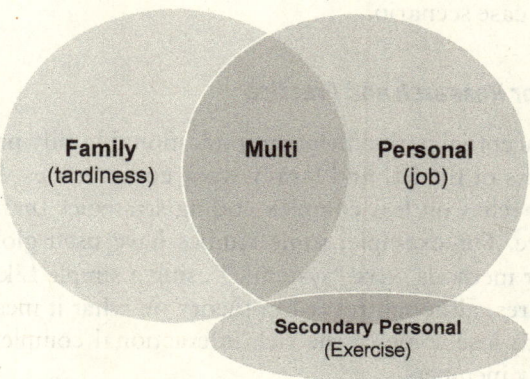

FIGURE 8.4. Graphic depiction of a secondary personal target behavior.

Summary of the Conceptual Model

Here, I advocate for recognition of the interdependence of change language. In the simplest of terms, here is the model I propose for reimagining change language in family work during conjoint sessions:

- *Principle 1.* Evoking change language from one individual should never lower the expression of the MI Spirit with other family members.
- *Principle 2.* Change talk is interdependent when working with groups of family members. An FTB involves actions from multiple family members. MTBs involve personal target behaviors that are closely related to the FTB.
- *Principle 3.* Evoking change talk for MTBs also builds motivation for the FTB. I propose calling this a multilevel change talk statement, which counts as change talk for a personal target behavior and a family-level one.
- *Principle 4.* Identifying MTBs when evoking change language for FTBs can yield broader benefits to families.
- *Principle 5.* When an individual has a secondary personal target behavior, it is one that has little or no relation to the FTB. Focusing on it in a family session would be distracting if the goal is to work on FTBs. Change talk about secondary personal target behaviors likely does not count toward the FTB.

Exercise 8.1 includes a practice activity for recognizing family-level ROARS skills, as well as identifying MTBs and FTBs. Use it to apply these principles to a case scenario.

Suggestions for Research and Practice

I hope this conceptualization helps spur additional family process research among members of the MI and family work communities. Family process research often relies on less complex coding strategies than the one I am suggesting here. For example, some studies have used global ratings on whether helper methods were "systemic" using a simple Likert scale. Such process measures, although rooted in theory on what it means to be "systemic," seem to lose some of the rich interactional complexities between different family members.

What remains unknown is how to aggregate the personal and family-level change talk into predictors of individual and family-level goals.

EXERCISE 8.1. Recognizing Family-Level and Multilevel Change Talk

Scenario: Bernard and Coco are seeking couples therapy.

Directions: Use the right column to label the helper's MI skills (reflection, open question, affirmation, and reflective summary), specifying whether they were at the individual or family level. For statements made by the couple, indicate if the statement is family-level or multilevel change talk.

HELPER: How about we start by you both telling me what you're hoping for from our time together?	
COCO: *(tearing up)* This is hard. We almost didn't come today. But we felt like, if we didn't, we were on a path toward divorce.	
HELPER: You are trying to figure out what's next for your relationship.	
BERNARD: We want to stay together if we can. It just seems like lots of things are tearing us apart.	
HELPER: That's the goal for you, Bernard. You have your reasons for working through this.	
BERNARD: I'm still in love with Coco and cannot imagine life without her, but some things have to change. I never imagined it would get this hard.	
HELPER: *(to Bernard)* It's a dark time, but for you, it's still worth it to stay together. *(to Coco)* And what are your thoughts, Coco?	
COCO: Same. I want to get back to a happier place and stay with Bernard.	
HELPER: *(to Bernard)* You're both in agreement that there is still something here worth saving, and you're both looking for help with some serious things that have been going on.	
COCO: Caring for a kid with a chronic health condition is draining all our energy. We love our son deeply, but we disagree on how to handle it.	
BERNARD: She's all work and kids.	
COCO: How can I not be?	
HELPER: *(to Bernard)* You both feel stuck in the pattern. You'd like her to spend more time with you, and *(to Coco)* you feel like if you let up things are going to fall apart.	
COCO: Yes, he's not super helpful with the kids.	
BERNARD: How can I be? They only want your help.	
HELPER: So, you both want to come to an agreement about how to handle your stress from parenting. You're both not happy and want something to change. This would improve your relationship. What else would improve if you were on the same page about parenting?	

THOUGHT QUESTIONS: (1) Why did the helper check to see if both partners wanted to stay together? (2) What is the family-level target behavior? (3) What may be some multilevel target behaviors that emerge later?

Individual level change talk, such as talking about getting to school on time, may reasonably predict family-level goal attainment. It would also be interesting to know if aggregate measures of all personal, multilevel, and family-level change talk predicted change, and for which target behaviors. That is, do each member's change talk statements, regardless of whether referring to one's specific behaviors or family-oriented goals, predict success in change? This hypothesis is reasonable, as recent work revealed that change talk among adolescents aggregated across all group members, predicted individual change (D'Amico et al., 2015).

For clinicians, focusing on eliciting interdependent motivations may be a highly salient way to engage families in thinking about their problems systemically through the framework of MI. The key takeaway here is that you can learn how to elicit and reinforce both individual and family-level change talk.

SUMMARY

In this chapter, I first defined family-level equipoise as even application of change talk generation across all family members who are present. Then, I noted how almost all current conceptualizations of change talk, even ones involving family members present, map onto one individuals' behavior change. To facilitate future practice and research innovations, I began outlining some principles for navigating the family-level and personal natures of change talk in working with multiple family members.

CHAPTER 9

Engaging Families with Motivational Interviewing

> No one cares how much you know
> until they know how much you care.
> —THEODORE ROOSEVELT

Engagement is the platform on which all successful helping relations rest (Miller & Rollnick, 2012), yet there is little rest for helpers engaging families. Mastering engagement takes energy. Sharp listening skills, attending to multiple relationships at once, and active leadership during initial sessions are required to successfully engage families. A large percentage of clients never return after the first session (Hamilton et al., 2011). The warm feel of MI, and its emphasis on resolving ambivalence, make it an attractive option for initial and early sessions.

Many family therapy texts outline key activities needed in the first few sessions (Nichols & Davis, 2020) or outline broad principles that make for effective practice (Gottman & Gottman, 2015; Sprenkle et al., 2009). Because this book aims to help practitioners integrate MI in family work, I only briefly discuss key tasks in engaging families. Then, I review how to balance engagement with family intake assessment activities. Next, I talk about how to sequence engagement, depending on whether the helper is starting with a whole family or an individual.

KEY TASKS IN ENGAGING FAMILIES

Nichols and Davis (2020) offer 10 important tasks to accomplish in the early phase of family work, including (1) engaging all members' perceptions of the family's problems and feelings about treatment; (2) leading and structuring the session; (3) being warm, yet professional; (4) identifying family strengths; (5) being empathic and respecting the family's autonomy; (6) focusing on specific problems and attempted solutions; (7) developing hypotheses about family interactions that maintain the problem and positive interaction that can combat it; (8) considering who else should be involved in treatment; (9) offering a treatment contract; and (10) inviting questions.

These activities in Nichols and Davis's (2020) text presume that all family members should be present in family work, diverging from this book's definition of family work. That is, I defined the key feature of family work as a systemic approach where helpers include more than one individual in treatment (see Chapter 1). In fact, there is limited agreement about who should be included in family work, with some advocating for everyone's presence and some arguing for the minimally sufficient network required to meet some therapeutic goal (Carr, 1990).

Later in the chapter, I discuss engagement when only one person or multiple people initially present for help. Let us first, however, tackle the issue of balancing engagement with initial assessment processes required in many settings.

Sequencing Engagement and Assessment

Helpers in most human service professions walk a tightrope between engagement and onerous agency paperwork processes. Often, there are funder mandates for completing assessments or initial treatment plans within a specified period. So just how does one listen intently, use two reflections for every question, and generate change talk when a diagnosis must be recorded in the first session?

Information collection can interrupt the flow of MI and its emphasis on reflective listening. This is especially true when asking various closed questions required to determine eligibility for services. One potential solution to this problem is to separate client engagement via MI from doing required eligibility assessments. Helpers proficient in MI often notice that assessment information collected on standardized intake forms can emerge organically through skilled listening. Structured and scientifically validated questionnaires are not without their merits. They sacrifice the client's narrative but can in return yield a trove of information that may inform practice (Smith & Hall, 2007). Such questions efficiently determine service

Combine client information from reflective listening with the information from assessments.

eligibility and allow for triaging clinical needs. Why not have the best of both worlds, combining client information from both traditions, the organic information arising from reflective listening and the clinical information from validated assessments?

In individually focused MI, there is an empirically validated method that balances engagement and assessment during an initial substance use assessment (Martino et al., 2006). The Motivational Interviewing Assessment: Supervisory Tools for Enhancing Proficiency (MIA-STEP) protocol introduced the concept of an MI "sandwich." The session begins with 20 minutes of MI, progresses to a structured agency assessment, and then ends with 20 more minutes of MI. In other words, rather than trying to intermingle MI with all the information-gathering questions on an agency assessment, this process allows MI to happen organically at the beginning and end of the session. This is important because information gathering questions are contraindicated in MI. It proves difficult to resolve ambivalence when you pepper someone with eligibility determination questions.

To my knowledge, there are only a few family-based assessment protocols that mimic the MIA-STEP process by integrating MI and standardized assessments at intake. Smith and Hall's (2007) Strengths-Oriented Referral for Teens (SORT) attempts to balance initial engagement with the need for collecting agency assessment information. This two-session assessment process involves both parents and teens presenting for substance use assessments to complete the Global Appraisal of Individual Needs, a comprehensive biopsychosocial assessment (Dennis et al., 2002). That is followed by an hour-long MI session that includes both the parent and teens to review the assessment. The helper meets with the teen for 20 minutes individually, then with the caregiver(s) individually for 20 minutes, and finally brings the family together for a conjoint discussion.

Recent adaptations of the Family Check-Up also integrate MI and assessment processes to enhance family engagement. The Family Check-Up involves completing both a structured assessment and is followed by a session using MI with parents (Berkel et al., 2021). Similarly, this model has been used with incarcerated adolescents and their parents (Slavet et al., 2005).

The key clinical principle in these models is that helpers can juxtapose MI with assessment processes. Collecting a dry assessment without any engagement may partially explain why some families choose to terminate treatment early. If your motivation wavers when you walk through the door, an intimidating agency assessment is unlikely to put you at ease. There is also perhaps a degree of autonomy respect in not subjecting individuals to multiple assessments immediately. That is, assessing for depression, trauma, substance dependence, family violence, infidelity, developmental problems, family conflict, and every other construct under the sun all at one time may compromise engagement for the sake of assessment efficiency. The MIA-STEP, SORT, and Family Check-Up models represent hybrid models that balance the collection of comprehensive assessments with client engagement. These models improved substance use treatment initiation among adolescents (Smith et al., 2009) and short-term engagement among adults (Carroll et al., 2006), respectively.

Change and Sustain Talk about Engagement

You cannot do much for people who don't engage in the helping process. Thus, examples in this chapter demonstrate how to use MI when the target behavior itself is engaging in family sessions. As noted earlier, change talk, then, is defined in these examples as any client statement in favor of treatment participation. As we know, sustain talk, the converse of change talk, occurs when clients verbalize statements against participation. The box below shows common sources of family member ambivalence about participation in treatment, which may materialize as sustain talk statements.

Common Reasons for Ambivalence about Participating in Family Work

- Fear of being scapegoated/triangulated
- Fear of family secrets being revealed
- Being overwhelmed from single parenting
- Viewing helpers as social control agents
- Intense family conflict
- Misunderstanding of family work processes
- Cultural mistrust
- Viewing the problem as an individual versus family problem

THOUGHT QUESTIONS: (1) In your future or current area of practice, what do you see as potential sources of ambivalence family members may have about participation in family work? (2) Which sources of ambivalence do you feel it is easier for you to accept as "legitimate" sources of ambivalence, and why?

Engagement: Pathways into Family Work

Figure 9.1 presents a flowchart that may be useful to helpers who integrate family members at various stages of the helping relationship. If you do full-fledged family therapy or couples therapy, and everyone presents together in initial sessions, you may consider the family unit as your client and insist on all members starting services simultaneously. Others who do family work may have services organized around a target client (a.k.a. identified client) who engages first, and then must engage other family members later. One possibility with that scenario is the challenge of dealing with both your identified client's ambivalence, as well as that of outside family members, of starting family sessions.

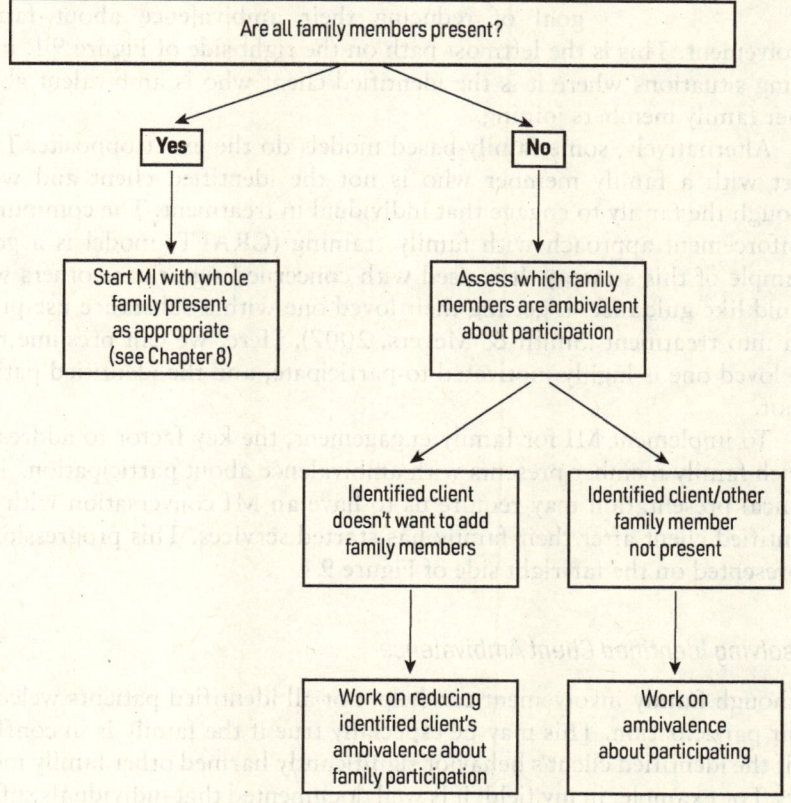

FIGURE 9.1. Engagement flowchart for family work.

Engaging Clients Individually

Some readers predominantly work with individuals and seek information about how to work through ambivalence toward participation in family work. There are a lot of different, and highly valid reasons, to start with the presenting client on an individual basis. Family members can be added later. For example, families differ in how much involvement they may want in an individual family member's treatment.

Two common situations exist where MI proves useful in engaging individual family members. First, helpers can talk to identified clients about including other family members. So, helpers may speak with the family members only after the identified client starts. In this situation, we could have an MI conversation with an identified client with the goal of reducing their ambivalence about family involvement. This is the leftmost path on the right side of Figure 9.1, indicating situations where it is the identified client who is ambivalent about other family members joining.

Which family member is ambivalent about participating?

Alternatively, some family-based models do the exact opposite. They start with a family member who is not the identified client and work through the family to engage that individual in treatment. The community reinforcement approach with family training (CRAFT) model is a good example of this strategy. It is used with concerned significant others who would like guidance in getting their loved one with a substance use problem into treatment (Smith & Meyers, 2007). Here, we can presume that the loved one is highly motivated to participate, and the identified patient is not.

To implement MI for family engagement, the key factor to address is which family member presents with ambivalence about participation. This clinical presentation may require us to have an MI conversation with the identified client after their family has started services. This progression is represented on the far-right side of Figure 9.1.

Resolving Identified Client Ambivalence

Although family involvement can help, not all identified patients welcome their participation. This may be especially true if the family is in conflict, or if the identified client's behavior significantly harmed other family members. For example, in my field, it is well documented that individuals suffering from addictions or risky substance use cause a lot of collateral damage to family and friends. Money is borrowed or stolen, promises are broken, and hurtful words are said. Yet, if it is ethically reasonable to encourage family participation, we can possibly mend some of those relationships, as well as work on the identified client's substance use. Importantly, we can treat client ambivalence about family participation in the same way we address other target behaviors, through expression of empathy, fostering collaboration, and generating change talk in reference to family participation (i.e., the target behavior).

Example: Identified Patient Reluctance for Family Involvement

Consider the following example where a client presenting with depression is discussing relationship problems with their fiancée. It is one of the top reasons that the client presented for treatment after being asked why they decided to come in for help in the first session. They feel their depression is affecting their loved one. Yet, ironically, the client feels ambivalent about integrating their partner into sessions. The helper is engaging the client, and they discuss involving their partner in family sessions.

CLIENT: I feel really distant from them right now and am worried about losing them because of how bad things have gotten.

HELPER: You don't want to lose them. That wouldn't do much for your depression. [Simple reflection]

CLIENT: Well, it would do a lot, but not in the right direction.

HELPER: And you want to move in the right direction, and you've taken an important step by coming here today. You had a small kernel of hope that coming here would get you out of your funk. [Complex reflection]

CLIENT: Yeah, but they just don't understand depression and take it personally when I'm not able to communicate how much I care about them.

HELPER: You would feel better if that improved, and you're feeling stuck about how to address that. So, what have you thought about doing, if anything? [Complex reflection, open question]

CLIENT: I got nothing.

HELPER: Could I make a suggestion? [Enhancing autonomy]

CLIENT: Sure.

HELPER: You can shoot it down if you don't like it. Sometimes, it has been helpful to clients with relationship problems to bring their partners in. There are a range of things we could do, if you're interested, like talking about strategies for improving communication. Or we could discuss what you're experiencing to help them understand more. Sometimes, partners feel that loved ones with depression aren't invested in the relationship, so family sessions may help them have more empathy and to see that your symptoms affect your communication with them. What are your thoughts? [Open question, enhancing partnership]

CLIENT: I'm not sure. I don't know if I'd have the energy to meet with both you and them. Sounds exhausting.

HELPER: The drain may not be worth it, and yet you really want to figure out how to make sure your depression doesn't endanger this relationship. [Complex reflection, double-sided]

CLIENT: Yes, things are bad.

HELPER: And you're just not sure that anything would come out of meeting with your partner and me together. [Complex reflection, amplification]

CLIENT: Could you tell me more about what we'd do if we all met together?

HELPER: You need some more details. I respect that. Even at your lowest, you're thinking about whether something is going to help move you one step closer to feeling better. You have so little energy from the depression. Everything is hard work, yet you persist. That's a hell of a place to be. [Affirmation, complex reflection]

CLIENT: You know your stuff. I've been to other providers that just didn't get this, or where I felt judged for not working "hard enough." (*Makes air quote signs with hands.*) I'm still not sure I'm ready to invite my partner in. Can we revisit this later when I have more energy?

HELPER: Absolutely. It seems like now is not the right time, and you're open to maybe trying this later at a time when you have a little more energy. Right now you feel you'd get more out of focusing on other pressing things. What is your top priority? [Complex reflection, open question, enhancing partnership]

A key consideration with MI is preserving the client's autonomy. MI is not foolproof prestidigitation that guarantees family engagement. We may or may not get all family members to the table, no matter how strong our desires are to work with multiple client systems. Yet, MI offers an effective tool for raising that conversation empathically when ambivalence about family participation exists.

Thus, MI is not a miracle salve for all therapeutic goals, such as the helper's desire to include the partner for systemic family work. In this situation, the goal was to explore the possibility of fiancée inclusion in sessions, via the strategy of expressing empathy and attempting to elicit change language around the target behavior of partner inclusion in the sessions. However, the client had other ideas. They ultimately communicated that it would involve mental strain to include their fiancée. This occurred despite efforts the helper made to elicit change language about partner involvement. When this happens, it is sometimes important to drop the pursuit of change talk at some point and focus on empathy and collaboration. That is, continuing to press for change talk here would undercut empathy. Careful attention to client statements aids engagement. Notice how even though there was sufficient sustain talk around family inclusion, the stage is set for client engagement on the target behavior of alleviating depression.

This short MI conversation also addresses multiple evidence-based strategies designed to boost overall client retention. McAdams and colleagues' (2018) systematic review identified six actionable strategies to boost family therapy retention, including (1) conveying understanding and support, (2) demonstrating knowledge and support, (3) communicating a genuine desire to help, (4) clearly describing the family therapy process, (5) communicating hope that problems can be resolved, and (6) creating a safe environment. In my view, the helper efficiently communicates both expertise and support through reflections about the nature of depression (i.e., "The drain may not be worth it . . . ") while also attending to processes thought to operate in MI to resolve ambivalence (i.e., evoking change talk). In that regard, the concept of multipurpose statements applies to engagement. That is, within the framework of MI, one can implement several of the common family therapy engagement strategies.

RESOLVING AMBIVALENCE OF FAMILY MEMBERS NOT INITIALLY PRESENT

The identified client may not be the only one with ambivalence about participation. In my work with families with adolescents, parents often want their kids to feel uninhibited in discussing their problems in individual sessions. These well-intentioned parents are often mindful of their teen's growing need for autonomy. However, one unfortunate byproduct of this is that they may overlook the benefits of family sessions and give the youth full veto power. In viewing this through an MI lens, it is critical to think of these situations on a case-by-case basis to form personalized reflections for such parents. Below is a brief dialogue example of engaging parents who are willing to be involved, but unsure if it would be helpful.

PARENT: We want to make sure they feel safe in therapy and that we aren't hindering any progress. [Sustain talk]

HELPER: So, you're really respectful of their autonomy, which you know is really important at this age. You're so thoughtful about parenting. [Reflection, affirmation]

PARENT: Yeah, it's so tough to know what to do . . . when to step in, when to back off.

HELPER: You think through each situation carefully. [Simple reflection] That's commendable. [Affirmation]

PARENT: Thanks. We're so overwhelmed right now. It's been tough.

HELPER: You're unsure what your role should be, and yet you want this helping relationship to work for them. [Complex reflection, double-sided]

PARENT: Yes, I feel like if we don't give them space it may not work.

HELPER: So, you may consider joining only if you have assurances that they have a lot of say about your involvement. It has to be timed right, and also not interrupt the relationship between your child and me. [Complex reflection, evocative]

PARENT: I see your point, but I think they need to feel safe to make progress.

HELPER: You have some reservations about involvement. Like I said, I think this comes from you being considerate. On the other hand, I'm curious if you could see any benefit from participating in sessions. In what ways would you and your child benefit if you sat in? [Reflection, evocative question]

For the sake of illustration, I ended this example at the point where some initial reflections and affirmations were used to establish empathy and collaboration, and the helper was transitioning to eliciting change talk. In this example, change talk would be in reference to parental participation in sessions. So, any statements parents made in the direction of session participation would constitute change talk, and those statements in favor of not participating would be sustain talk. It is easy to see how this discussion could achieve some of the early engagement tasks suggested in family work. For example, through the course of generating change talk in this conversation, the helper could keep an eye out for family strengths, interaction patterns, and past attempted solutions to problems faced by the family. Family engagement is one among several processes in MI, and they are not strange bedfellows.

I've also encountered parents that seemed so disengaged from their kids and who felt like the responsibility for behavior change rested squarely on the youth. Obviously, that scenario conflicts with reframing difficulties as systemic family problems. In youth work, helpers sometimes label these parents as ones that just want to "drop off their kids for us to fix." This cognitive framing by clinicians captures genuine frustrations about parents who elude engagement.

Yet, the label is not helpful if we're to successfully engage parents. Such statements are said by helpers who are blowing off steam. Yet, these negative statements about parents made by helpers are also value statements about the important role of families in child rearing and solving problems. Thus, helpers need to consider the parent's perspective to communicate empathy. For example, sometimes disengaged parents are also hindered by a deep distrust of the social service system due to perceived systematic discrimination. Such parents present a challenge for integration into family work, but it is possible for helpers to reframe parental reluctance to engage in sessions as naturally occurring ambivalence. Consider the following example of a parent that is asked to meet with a social worker after her teenage child got caught shoplifting.

HELPER: And how do you feel about coming in and chatting about how you can support LaShonda? [Open question]

PARENT: She's grown. She's gotta make her own choices now. [Sustain talk]

HELPER: You've tried hard as a parent, and now want them to take some responsibility. [Complex reflection]

PARENT: Yes, and with all due respect to you, I don't like social workers. They're just in it for a check. [Sustain talk]

HELPER: You've had some bad experiences with my kind. You got some scars from that. [Complex reflection, empathy]

PARENT: Yes, always up in my business. I'm doing the best I can. I can't get ahead if I have to keep meeting with you people. You might as well be the police. [Sustain talk]

HELPER: You've had a lot of struggles. It's like the powers that be are working against you and not on your behalf. It makes you angry. [Complex reflection, empathy]

PARENT: Hell, yes, I'm angry. How would you feel if you couldn't make ends meet, had gangs running wild in your back yard, could get shot by the cops for doing nothing, and got people telling you where to go every damn hour of your day. "Go get a job, go get to your probation officer, go sign up for this class, talk to this person about your kid. . . ." And you come in here with your nice clothes and that smile.

Helper: It's hard to make sense out of all of this. So much pain that you don't see any benefits of talking with me about your kid. [Complex reflection, empathy]

Parent: I can barely take care of my own self.

Helper: You keep going even though you got it bad. [Simple reflection] That takes a lot of strength. [Affirmation]

Parent: I suppose.

Helper: And you're not sure this is the right way to go about it, yet you want your kid to have it better than you did. [Complex reflection, evoking change talk]

Parent: You got that right. All I can think is that it gets a little better every generation.

Helper: It all hurts, and maybe there is just some part of you that thinks it can get better for you and LaShonda. [Complex reflection, empathy]

Parent: You got to think that. Otherwise, you'd have no hope.

Helper: You just put one foot in front of the other in the face of hard things. That takes guts. If we were to keep working together, what could I do, if anything, to help? [Reflection, open question, enhancing partnership]

Here, notice a few things. First, there is always temptation to engage in discussion about current events, especially if you see them in a different light from the client. Whatever your feelings about systemic discrimination, police violence, or whether a client is trying hard enough as a parent, empathy can only be communicated if you attempt to step into your client's shoes. Second, an additional pitfall may ensnare some helpers who feel compelled to directly argue with the client's statement that her teenage daughter is grown up. That client statement seems to signal an abdication of parental responsibility. Arguing that point, however, may set up an antagonistic relationship and sacrifice empathy. Arguing with a client in this manner exemplifies what is known in the MI community as the *fixing reflex*, or the tendency to want to make "right" something you see as wrong from your point of view. However, fixing it by arguing the point would likely result in more sustain talk and a ruptured relationship. Finally, I'm often asked whether I think reflecting back some client statements borders on condoning their behavior. For example, the target behavior here is parental involvement, so how do we not send a message that reinforces parental disengagement. The short answer is that the dual focus of empathy and cultivating change talk work well to do that. You have to start with empathy in tense situations like the one above. That is, the helper is simultaneously reflecting the statement back about how the parent is feeling about participation (i.e., "She's grown. She gotta make her own choices now"), while keeping an eye on parental involvement in their program. Although the reasons for the parental disengagement (i.e., violence, hopelessness, perceived discrimination) are met with empathy, there is no statement that directly condones it. Instead, at the end of the interaction there is a gentle nudge toward involvement in additional sessions where the door may be open to further address parenting and things this parent can do to help her daughter.

> Empathy can only be communicated if you attempt to step into your client's shoes.

Additional Example of Engaging a Reluctant Family Member

Family therapists worry about triangulation, or having some combination of the family members, and possibly the helper, siding against one individual. Helpers from the MI tradition should respect the autonomy of individuals that have justifiable ambivalence about joining family therapy for fear of being triangulated. On the other hand, as systemic thinkers, this doesn't preclude using MI to resolve ambivalence in clients about either (1) adding family members to work with identified patients or (2) adding straggling members to family-based treatments.

In this latter situation, it may be beneficial to discuss with the first wave of family members arriving to treatment about the need to respect the autonomy of a family member yet to join. Sometimes, you simply must focus on what can be accomplished without them present. Further, if that straggling member feels pressure from other family members it may overwhelm them and result in more sustain talk, this time in response to family members. If straggling family members are fed up with their families pressuring them to join, one possibility is that a helper can call them. Below is an example of how such a conversation may sound.

HELPER: Thanks for agreeing to speak with me about your possibly joining the rest of your family to work with me. [Autonomy respect from "possibly joining" qualifier]

RELUCTANT FAMILY MEMBER: I know what this is all about. All of them are going to sit around and tell me what I'm doing wrong.

HELPER: You may be willing to do this, but you need to know that you'll be heard... that the rest of your family isn't going to shine a spotlight on you. [Complex reflection, empathic and evocative]

RELUCTANT FAMILY MEMBER: Yeah, that sums it up.

HELPER: Their ganging up on you would be very hurtful. [Complex reflection, empathy]

RELUCTANT FAMILY MEMBER: It's downright hypocritical. Nobody's hands are clean in this family. I've got my things, but they have theirs, too.

HELPER: So, it sounds like you're trying to avoid being attacked and feeling a lot of pressure. [Simple reflection, empathy]

RELUCTANT FAMILY MEMBER: Yes, it's just not fair that I'm always the black sheep. My family is always telling me, "You did that," "You are making all of us miserable," "You are never going to be anything."

HELPER: It hurts. [Simple reflection, empathic]

RELUCTANT FAMILY MEMBER: Yeah. I'm so angry.

HELPER: And you never get anywhere right now with expressing your anger. It never changes how they see you. You want that to change. [Complex reflection, evocative]

RELUCTANT FAMILY MEMBER: I don't know. We may be too far gone.

HELPER: You don't think things will ever get better between all of you. [Complex reflection, amplification]

RELUCTANT FAMILY MEMBER: I wouldn't go that far. It's just gonna take a lot of work and time. You know... time heals all.

HELPER: So, a small part of you could see a future where you all get along. [Simple reflection, using tentative language]

RELUCTANT FAMILY MEMBER: Yeah, I guess I'm not ready to give up.

HELPER: How would that be better for you if things got better with your family? [Simple reflection, evocative]

ENGAGING FAMILIES

When multiple family members are present, principles discussed earlier apply. That is, pivoting attention between family members is required to hear all perspectives. Keep family-level equipoise in mind. As previously discussed, this involves not using some MI skills that benefit one individual and offend other family members.

All family members' perceptions about the treatment process should be assessed. That is, are some family members more or less eager about seeing you? Was somebody dragged to your office and doing this to get out of hot water with other family members? **Split alliances** occur in family work when helpers have stronger alliances with certain members and weaker ones with others. Split alliances negatively impact outcomes (Friedlander et al., 2018). So, it is critical that helpers reflect upon whether or not they have stronger working alliances with some members rather than others. The box below discusses a situation in my work where conditions were ripe for developing a split alliance. The bottom line is that helpers should reflect on whether they feel stronger affinities for certain family members, so they can remember to demonstrate empathy with the others present.

Look out for split alliances.

"What about Javier?"

Early in my training, I took a family therapy practicum course where students saw real families. Teams of two to four students took turns running sessions. Students not in the session, as well as the instructor, observed the session from behind a double-sided mirror and had the capability to send a suggestion to the helpers via earbuds they wore in the session.

The family I was assigned to was a couple where Javier was approximately 20 years older than his female partner, Jane. They were a moderately distressed couple with commonly occurring communication problems such as not feeling appreciated by each other, as well as role conflicts regarding home maintenance and child raising responsibilities. Over time, it occurred to us that we felt more sympathy for Jane. Javier was viewed by some student therapists as exhibiting some toxic masculinity behaviors. Thus, that made him a villain in their family story.

By reflecting on this in our team supervision, we identified that we should keep an eye on our therapeutic alliance with Javier, lest we communicate more empathy for Jane. Sympathy and repulsion are normally occurring feelings for all helpers, but *empathy* is a verb in MI.

THOUGHT QUESTIONS: (1) What values do you hold that would incline you to side with one family member over another in some situations? (2) What would some signs be for you that this was happening? (3) How could you preserve or repair your relationship with the individual with whom you don't identify as strongly?

Need for Orientation (a.k.a. Ground Rules)

Several things not typically considered to be part of MI proper should transpire in early sessions. For example, helpers need to discuss whether they allow one member to speak confidentially to them about behaviors that affect other family members. Examples include discussions about infidelity, substance use, or other behaviors that may embarrass individuals and send shockwaves through already shaky relationships. Outlining such policies is important, as it may place some limits on client autonomy, which is a central MI concept.

FAMILY ENGAGEMENT AND SOCIAL JUSTICE

Fifty years ago, helpers described the ideal client as young, attractive, verbal, intelligent, and successful (YAVIS), which in this era seems like thinly veiled and coded language for middle-class White clientele (Schofield, 2019). Now, it is increasingly more common to read discussions of considering power dynamics due to therapist's oftentimes privileged backgrounds, and all major professional helping organizations including diversity as a value in their codes of ethics (Knudson-Martin et al., 2019; McDowell et. al., 2019; Seedall et al., 2014). Helpers simply must reflect upon whether client marginalization due to sexism, racism, classism, homophobia or other mechanisms affects engagement.

There is increasing attention to cultural adaptation of MI. Lee's (2025) volume provides a strong rationale for adapting MI to be more culturally relevant and provides some practical guidance. Research studies show that such cultural adaptations are effective for Latino immigrants (Lee et al., 2011), African Americans, and Native Americans (Venner et al., 2006; D'Amico et al., 2020). Additionally, meta-analytic reviews reveal that effect sizes for MI with ethnic minority clients are about double those observed for White clients (Hettema et al., 2005).

There remains a lot of debate about how to reduce health disparities among ethnic minorities, including premature exits from therapy. Some have advocated diversifying the workforce so that the helping staff in social services and medicine represent the populations they serve, which increases client comfort, but racial/ethnic matching of clients and helpers has not translated into better clinical outcomes (Cabral & Smith, 2011). Others suggest that cultural adaptation of programs would be the best route, as some evidence suggests there are indeed better outcomes (Benish et al., 2011). Implementation difficulties, however, may exist in areas where there are not high concentrations of ethnic minority clients and adapted approaches only apply to a certain percent of one's clientele. Finally, a third option for addressing cultural competence involves increasing cultural humility through provision of MI (Windsor et al., 2018). That is, some argue that MI's heavy emphasis on active listening and empathy is, in essence, culturally competent by default. You cannot be empathic without conveying an understanding of how one's social background may be contributing to their problems.

It may even be that some reflections deliberately tap into cultural themes, validating client's lived experiences in a multicultural world. My colleagues and I have referred to such reflections as **culturally accurate reflections** (Windsor et al., 2018). These may be especially important when engaging families. These reflections are based on strong guesses by the helper based on knowledge of cultural groups values, as well as in-depth listening. For example, a culturally accurate reflection to a religious African American family may be "Faith is where you find your community." Alternatively, in Latino families, there are sometimes strong *machismo* and *familismo* values, where the former refers to hypermasculinity and the latter refers to the valuing families over individuals. Thus, a culturally accurate reflection to a lower-income middle-aged Latino immigrant may emphasize his perceptions of masculinity and family values: "You are working so hard to support your family and it is difficult to watch your son become more Americanized and spend so much time away from you." Naturally, one must remember to be mindful of intragroup diversity. Do not assume that all members of a particular group share the same values.

An MI Caveat

In our exuberance to right the wrongs of diminished access to therapy among individuals from ethnic minority backgrounds, it would be remiss not to discuss potential harms that can be done via well-intentioned professionals. Could it be that sometimes being compassionate means that you accept the families' right not to engage in treatment, even when such treatment appears relevant to ethnic minorities' presenting problems? Could family engagement involve a dangerous dance with criminal justice-related sanctions in some contexts?

Like it or not, social and other health services providers often serve a social control function. Sometimes, parents are required to attend mandatory classes prior to divorce or at the bequest of the child welfare system. Failure to attend could result in consequences.

In December 2020, Kenneth Bourne II, a social worker in Philadelphia, wrote an opinion piece entitled, "Shaming Exhausted Parents for their Kids' School Attendance Issues is Misguided and Unfair." In it, he described a single African American mother of four that was working multiple jobs and didn't know how to set up a Chromebook for her child. Simply expressing compassion via affirmations was the key that unlocked the family engagement door.

This story contains a cautionary tale for family workers. Is it possible that requiring some forms of family engagement may in some situations disproportionately burden parents from lower socioeconomic backgrounds? Are family engagement policies or required attendance systematically stressing already overwhelmed families? So, an ethical question for family workers is how to provide systemic treatments that do not create conditions that systematically exacerbate the disproportionate representation of racial/ethnic minorities in the legal system.

EVALUATING ENGAGEMENT

Family workers should tune into statements in favor of participation in family work as a key signal of engagement. We conceptualize these pro-change statements about participating in family work as change talk, and statements about reluctance to join the rest of the family as sustain talk. A gradual weakening of sustain talk, and an increase in change talk, provides a barometer of engagement. Part of learning MI involves evaluating the subtleties of change talk and sustain talk, to guide transitions from talking about why engagement may benefit the client toward collaboratively conceptualizing a plan of action. Exercise 9.1 presents a practice activity for recognizing and responding to change language about session participation.

Another method for evaluating engagement is simply whether the clients vote with their feet. Did they return for additional sessions? If so, engagement can be evaluated during all interactions with clients. Within the change talk/sustain talk framework, you can continually reevaluate your clients' ambivalence at all stages of the helping relationship. Many helpers understand that some clients show up to sessions and seem to be just going through the motions rather than doing therapeutic work. We will talk about other stages of the helping relationship in the next chapter.

Finally, the degree to which clients agree that systemic family work will ameliorate their troubles, may be a particularly relevant type of change talk to heed. According to Wampold and Imel (2015), three main components

EXERCISE 9.1. Evaluating Family Member Engagement

Instructions: For client statements, underline change talk. Circle portions of the statement that may constitute sustain talk. In the box on the right, imagine that you are the helper and formulate a reply that either (1) reflects back the client statement empathically, (2) nudges on or reinforces change talk in reference to engagement, or (3) accomplishes both (i.e., a multipurpose reflection).

Client statement	Helper response
1. *Example:* "<u>I may be willing to come,</u> (but only if they don't throw stones my way.)"	*Example:* "If you felt safe, there may be some benefits to you in going."
2. "I'm in. Seems like you're willing to give me cover and make sure they don't gang up on me."	
3. "No way. Look, I'm willing to chat with you one on one a bit, but I'm not coming to a family session. That'll be a bloodbath."	
4. "I guess I'll come if it will make my partner happy."	
5. "I just don't see how meeting as a family will help them. They need to do this by themselves."	
6. "I'm willing to come and give it a shot."	
7. "This sounds great. I really think this will give us a platform to talk about things we usually avoid as a family. I cannot wait to get started."	

drive therapeutic outcomes: (1) common factors such as the relationship with the helper, (2) myth acceptance, and (3) the actual content of the services (i.e., communication skills training, relapse prevention programming). Myth acceptance (discussed in Chapter 3) is defined as the shared language system between helper and client about what methods will lead to reductions of one's problems. For example, if clients agree that all members of the family are affected by a problem and all must contribute to its resolution, they share in the myth of systemic family work. The *myth* provides the framework for thinking about the problem and instills hope about problem resolution. Selectively reinforcing client change talk in later sessions about myth acceptance over time may instill hope about family work.

Simply monitoring change talk and session attendance, however, is not always foolproof. I recently met with a client at the beginning of a second session who told me that I was easy to talk to and that he felt I listened to him and didn't judge him. What excellent examples of change talk surrounding engagement! He was referred to me by his partner, who wanted him to eliminate drinking entirely. He reported a past history of alcoholism, and in the recent past his consumption was two to three drinks per day, which enraged his partner. The client did not see eye to eye with his partner on the abstinence goal. He also didn't relate to members of 12-step fellowships like Alcoholics Anonymous. He talked about bringing in his partner for a future session, and he also wanted to explore the use of medications for addressing his alcohol use. After this second session with me, and subsequently receiving a prescription for anti-anxiety medications, I never saw him again. I would have liked to have done some systemic family work with him, but he had other plans. I hope that this brief encounter with me set him on a path toward improving his relationship with his partner.

One of my mentors used to tell me that, if you only have a hammer, all your clients start looking like nails. So, if you have beds to fill in your residential treatment center, do you become biased toward filling them? If you mainly do systemic work, do you show disdain for families that do not buy in? What I like about MI is that it encourages me to look at a broad number of routes by which people can heal, including only brief interactions with me that don't fit the traditional definition of engaging in services.

SUMMARY

Family engagement is about setting the stage for a productive helping relationship. Here, I reviewed one common problem in family work: lack of participation by family members whose presence may improve outcomes.

Engaging Families with MI

Through empathic communication and fostering change talk about participation, some family members may elect to participate. When family members elect not to participate, respecting their autonomy may be challenging.

Engaging can create a positive first impression of the helper, instilling hope. Helpers continue to engage families throughout the helping relationship. Other important tasks also produce positive outcomes for families. We will turn our attention to these tasks in the chapter that follows.

CHAPTER 10

Focusing, Evoking, and Planning in Family Work

> The secret of getting ahead is getting started. The secret of getting started is breaking your complex, overwhelming tasks into small manageable tasks, and then starting on the first one.
> —Mark Twain

You have raised the family's hopes that working with you will be fruitful. You've convinced them that you listen well, understanding their basic dilemmas. You've carefully attended to each person, so nobody feels like a scapegoat. By actively listening, you have some nebulous picture of their various goals, even if they haven't said them out loud. After all, you do have years of training. With ideas congealing on what you may offer the family, you possess a basic understanding of who is most ambivalent about engaging in treatment and familial conflicts.

Now what? You wouldn't want to leave your health care provider's office without actionable steps to alleviate some malady you're experiencing. So, it also goes with family work. Engagement is the first, and foundational, step in family work. After engaging families, we proceed with identifying what problems families most want resolved and what activities they are willing to do to resolve them. Miller and Rollnick (2012, 2023) referred to these tasks as focusing, evoking, and planning. Together with engaging, these concepts are collectively referred to as the four tasks of MI. We addressed engagement in Chapter 9, as it pertained to bringing family members into the fold. As we will see here, we never really stop engaging families. In this chapter, I use a single case example to illustrate the use of focusing, evoking, and planning.

Focusing, Evoking, and Planning in Family Work

Stage or process theories are useful heuristics to outline the general processes in family work. Yet, we must avoid the trap of thinking that they move linearly, with no overlap between concepts. For example, collaborative goal selection, although technically filed under focusing or planning in Miller and Rollnick's (2023) four-tasks model, may also reinforce engagement. Goals are even uttered by clients during the initial engagement, even if the helper believes they still need to continue developing rapport. This comes as no surprise, considering that one of the first questions used to start clinical encounters is often a variation of, "Tell me a little bit about why you're here."

In the box below I reflect on an experience observing a helper getting stuck in these four tasks. The key point is that you may find yourself cycling through engaging, evoking, planning, or focusing activities all in

---

"I Can't Help Them. They're in Precontemplation!"

Rigid use of concepts can derail treatment, including trying to lay treatment out as if it were a tidy linear process with engagement complete by session one, a collaborative treatment plan forged in session two, and implementation and troubleshooting done in sessions three through eight. This chapter applies three of Miller and Rollnick's (2012) four tasks to family work, including focusing, evoking, and planning. I see a lot of heuristic value in these concepts yet wonder if rigid application of such heuristics could potentially prove iatrogenic.

For example, as a clinical supervisor, I have heard clinicians refer to clients they perceived as nonresponsive to treatment as being stuck in precontemplation, the first and most ambivalence-ridden stage of Prochaska and DiClemente's (1982) transtheoretical model of change. What bothered me is that the label seemed to carry some negative energy in terms of clinicians feeling that they had done all they could do until clients were ready to change. The statement appeared to be salve for the clinician's insecurities at the cost of movement for the client. This possibly signaled frustration with not moving on beyond initial engagement.

I wonder if the trouble may have arisen due to thinking that one could end engagement and move on to treatment planning at a specified time. Consider the potential for zigging and zagging through the tasks when various clinical duties arise.

THOUGHT QUESTIONS: (1) What is your comfort level for how long engagement should last? (2) Have you ever been to a health care provider who gave you a treatment plan with little input from you? What was your reaction?

the same session. I illustrate such a session here. Also, if as described in this box, you find yourself labeling a client as not ready to change, consider what the four tasks described below may offer on how to proceed.

Switching between engagement, evoking, focusing, and planning requires careful timing based on the cues families provide. For example, rushing to solve problems families do not think they have is often referred to as the **premature focus trap**. In fact, rushing to solutions can jeopardize your relationship with families, hurting engagement. On the other hand, we also must acknowledge that some helpers may lean toward a **superfluous engagement trap**. A superfluous engagement trap would be where a helper stays stuck only in engagement. It involves a reluctance to moving on toward co-creating helpful solutions with families, even when all cues indicate that the family is ready. In other words, superfluous engagement happens when the family is ready to move faster than the clinician on planning solutions to their problems. Both traps signal lower empathy because they indicate that a helper is not accurately understanding the client perspective. Paying attention to the family's change and sustain language can guide helpers to know how quickly to continue through the tasks.

Both superfluous engagement and premature focus signal lower empathy.

FOCUSING

Simply put, focusing involves putting some parameters on helping conversations. In other words, what will you work on with the client? At times, this is somewhat prescribed by your area of specialization. For example, if you work in child protection, your chief goal involves preventing child abuse and neglect. Easy right? Well, not if we consider the sundry reasons families come to the attention of the system and their multiple needs. Focusing involves narrowing down the purpose of the helping relationship, including triaging the family's immediate needs.

In keeping with the spirit of collaboration, some MI practitioners start with a menu of options under the general rubric of the agency mission, allowing the family to choose its course within a certain range. Clients, like drivers using global positioning systems (GPS) to travel, sometimes pick different paths. Yet, the destination is the same whether we take the family or helper's route. First, however, you must know the destination. That is exactly what focusing is about.

The destination is the same whether we take the family or helper's route.

Focusing, Evoking, and Planning in Family Work

Consider the following conversation with a couple that lost custody of their child due to maternal substance use and paternal incarceration. The helper engaged the couple, affirming their strength and perseverance through a difficult situation. They processed anger toward the child welfare system and bypassed reluctance about seeing a court-mandated counselor via unrelenting empathy. Now comes the time to focus on the roadmap toward change.

HELPER: So, as you think about everything that's going on, and everything the court is asking you to do, what would you like to tackle first? [Open question, evocation, collaboration]

MOTHER: I think the drugs are the first thing that have to change.

FATHER: And I really need a job.

HELPER: You're both committed to getting your son back, and getting a job and getting off drugs are two ways to move closer to that. [Family-level complex reflection, reinforcing change talk]

FATHER: She's right. They hate moms on drugs. Freaks them the hell out. We may not be one of them perfect television families, but we love our kid. That's what they don't get.

HELPER: You both hate being judged for your family's problems. It doesn't mean that you aren't trying your hardest to be good parents. [Family-level complex reflection, empathy]

MOTHER: (*tearing*) Yes. I know I'm messed up. But our kid is still better off with us than some stranger.

HELPER: You're at a breaking point, and him being in foster care is unthinkable. Now, the task is just trying to figure out how to do that. What would be a good first step for you regarding the drug use? [Complex reflection, open question, focusing]

Notice in this example, that reinforcing change language does not end after you've started focusing. Even in a conversation that started on defining treatment goals, the helper rotates back and forth between reinforcing change language, maintaining a relationship through affirmations, and continuing to inquire about next steps. There is a fluidity of these tasks. Here, we see elements of engagement, evocation, and focusing. This snippet is evocative because the roadmap to change is being elicited from the family. Also, engagement is enhanced through affirmations and the warm feel of the statements (e.g., reflections). The clients continue to voice sadness and anger about their predicament. It would be ill-advised not to address such emotional content, even as the helper wants to move toward bringing goals into focus. In fact, as noted above, the phenomenon of a rush toward solutions at the expense of empathy has a name, the **premature focus trap.** Here, it is focusing because there are two different specific steps defined by the family in how they want to proceed with changing. These steps included getting a job and getting off drugs, which were voiced by the family in response to the helper asking, "What would you like to tackle first?"

In a way, focusing applies the same principles of cognitive-behavioral therapy to the helping relationship itself. You can see how larger goals are broken down into small measurable tasks all in the context of defining the helping relationship. Setting goals is critically important because goal setting is related to clinical outcomes. It is considered so critical that a recent systematic review identified over 104 different measures of goal setting (Lloyd et al., 2019).

EVOKING

As goals start to take shape, let us turn our attention to the evocation task. As previously defined, evocation is almost the exact opposite of doling out expert prescriptions for change. Instead, helpers use MI to draw out clients' wisdom and preferences for routes to change. Furthermore, evocation continually addresses motivation by keeping one eye on change talk, even while continuing to bring goals and treatment tasks to focus. Let's pick up where we left off in our example, and address autonomy issues that arise when clients are not thrilled with external pressure to change.

MOTHER: Well, I have to do residential treatment to get him back.

HELPER: And you're not crazy about that idea, but you're willing to go through with it because you're determined. [Complex reflection, empathy, and reinforcing change talk]

MOTHER: Exactly. I'm not gonna learn anything new in treatment I don't already know. I'm just doing it now to check a box. I've been to treatment three times.

HELPER: You want some permanent change now in your substance use. (*Pivoting to father.*) And what do you think about her going to treatment? [Reflection, open question]

FATHER: I mostly agree with her, except that she's gotta get through the dopesick phase.

HELPER: So, you see some benefits of residential with helping through withdrawals, and (*to mother*) perhaps you do, too. [Family-level reflection, change talk]

MOTHER: That's one good thing about treatment.

HELPER: It may give you a boost to make it on the outside after that. [Simple reflection, reinforcing change talk]

MOTHER: That's where it counts.

HELPER: And you both want this badly because your family will be better off. How else will you two benefit if you make changes in your drug use? [Family level reflection and family-level open question]

FATHER: It's gonna take me a while to get on my feet. Nobody hires felons.

HELPER: So, you see her getting sober as helping the family financially while you work your way up. [Reflection, reinforcing change talk]

FATHER: Yeah.

MOTHER: We've talked about that. He may even do some of the child care while I'm working if he cannot find anything good.

HELPER: So, you may have some financial benefits, too. What else? [Reflection, open question, evoking change talk]

MOTHER: So many things. I want to feel better. I want my kid back. I'd like us to be able to buy a house eventually.

FATHER: Yes (*nodding*).

HELPER: Your dreams are on hold until you do something about the drugs. And in a perfect world, if you didn't have to go to residential treatment, what would you two do next? [Complex reflection, reinforcing change talk, family-level open question, planning]

FATHER: I'd probably keep her at home for a whole week and watch her. That way, I'd know she wasn't going out to score.

HELPER: (*to father*) You're both in this together, and you're willing to step up your game if you have to. (*to mother*) And I imagine that you feel lucky to have a partner willing to do this for you. [Family-level and individual reflections, reinforcing change talk]

The helper has started to bring target behaviors into focus. During this evoking task, the parents indicate that the roadmap to the ultimate family level target behavior of family reunification starts with two other intermediary steps. In the conceptualization of family change talk I presented earlier, the mom's drug use and father's job seeking are both multilevel target behaviors. They are both individual target behaviors, but they map onto the family level target behavior of family reunification. Evoking can bring to light the big picture and identify the next steps needed to achieve the family's ultimate goal. Evoking is especially important for complex behavior changes.

Here, evocation refers both to the systematic elicitation and reinforcement of change talk surrounding goal importance (i.e., finances, reunification, buying a house), as well as the initial inquiry to evoke a potential plan to reduce drug use. Recall that change talk does not exist in a vacuum. It is always in relation to a target behavior. With reduced ambivalence and increased focus, a target behavior could be synonymous with a goal. For example, if a client has decided to get a job, any language in the direction of that target behavior would be considered change talk. For example, if the client said, "I could call that place that matches temporary employees with jobs," it would be considered change talk. This could be said in response to an evocative question like "What would you like to try to get a job?" However, lower evocation here would consist of the helper defining a plan before seeking input from the client (e.g., "I'd like you to consider calling the employment agency today").

> Change talk does not exist in a vacuum. It is linked to a specific target behavior.

Some helpers may be uncomfortable with the plan this couple articulated. There are some safety considerations, such as medical complications from withdrawal and the feasibility of the plan to consider. Yet, directly challenging the plan could potentially pop the motivation balloon into which the helper breathed some life. After all, the commonly used measure of therapeutic alliance, the Working Alliance Inventory, contains myriad items about the client/helper concordance on goals (Horvath & Greenberg, 1989). Furthermore, goal consensus between client and helpers predicts psychotherapy outcomes (Tryon et al., 2018).

Professional expertise and client selected goals need not collide. But finesse, rather than brute force communication, may be required. This means avoiding confrontational or paternalistic messages that convey helpers are the experts who unyieldingly impart their wisdom. Instead, and in keeping with the underlying spirit of MI, helpers attempt to use such instances to communicate collaboration, autonomy, and compassion.

> Your expertise and the client's goals need not collide.

Some strategies that may be useful for collaboratively developing a plan that integrates both professional expertise and clients' strengths include (1) asking clients how confident they are that they can implement the plan using either a scaling or open question, (2) asking permission to give advice about professional concerns (e.g., medical complications, experiences with other clients not successfully implementing the plan), (3) asking if they have any alternative ideas in addition to the plan, or (4) asking how they think the plan would meet expectations by the referral source.

Of course, despite my repeated use of the word "asking" here, please recall that reflections may achieve all these purposes and check some other boxes, too, such as both conveying empathy and addressing aspects of the change plan all at the same time. I referred to these types of statements as **multipurpose statements**. Look for opportunities to use reflections to achieve the same purpose as some of these questions I've listed above that are designed to handle potential discordance between the helper and client on goal selection.

PLANNING

In planning, our central task is to identify how the family wants to go about making changes. We transition from "why" they should change (i.e., engaging, evoking), "what" should change (i.e., focusing), and address the "how" of change. As you can see in the case example we've been using, sometimes there is substantial overlap in these tasks. Let us revisit what planning may look like with this couple.

HELPER: So, you both are considering some major changes, (*to mother*) you wanting to work on substance use, and (*to father*) you wanting to work on a job. You're heartbroken that your kid is not with you and so you're determined to do these things [Family-level complex reflection]. Now, I wonder how you plan to go about this. What would work for you? [Open evocative question]

MOTHER: Like I said, I need treatment. I need to kick. But there's gonna be a waiting list.

HELPER: That's frustrating. Waiting is messing with you, and you wanna do this now. [Reflection, empathy, reinforcing change talk]

MOTHER: Yeah, it's like I cannot catch a break.

HELPER: One more thing, and yet you're pretty tough. [Double-sided reflection]

MOTHER: Yeah, I can get through the waiting-list period.

HELPER: I'm wondering how you two will do this together. What are both your thoughts? [Family-level open question]

FATHER: Well, we can check and see if you can do outpatient until a bed opens up.

MOTHER: Yeah, I suppose.

HELPER: It's not what you want, yet you may be willing to do it. Or perhaps you have other ideas? [Double sided reflection, empathy, reinforcing change talk, open question]

MOTHER: I think I may like to try the medications that reduce cravings.

HELPER: That's a great idea. [Affirmation]

FATHER: Isn't that just substituting one drug for another. I'm not sure I like that. [Sustain talk in relation to mother's multilevel target behavior]

HELPER: You're worried that it won't work, and that scares you. You're desperate for her to get better. [Complex reflection, empathy]

FATHER: I mean . . . I've heard it's no better than being high and that people sell that shit. So, it's gotta be addictive.

HELPER: And you want whatever approach you two choose to not just be another addiction. [Simple reflection, empathy] Like substituting one addiction for another. I'm wondering what else you know about the medications, and also if it would be helpful to you to share what I know. Choice is still up to you. Maybe I can just help you make an informed choice. [Enhancing autonomy and partnership]

MOTHER AND FATHER: (*Nod.*)

HELPER: So, there are a couple of options. Methadone is the oldest one and a lot of studies say it works. What is does is provide a lower safer dose to help manage cravings. It is closely monitored, and clinics will often limit how much they give you. The downside is sometimes you have to make a lot of trips. They will give you more doses to take home after you've attended a while or submitted negative urine tests for other opioids. Suboxone is another option. That one is something that can be taken orally, like if you've ever seen those breath mint films that melt in your mouth. It combines two different drugs to help with cravings. Both contain opioids, but when used as prescribed and with other treatment and social support can be effective.

FATHER: So, you're telling me the only way to get off opioids is to use opioids. That just don't seem right.

HELPER: (*to father*) I hear your concerns loud and clear, and (*to mother*)

I'm also wondering what your thoughts are. [Reflection, empathy, open question]

MOTHER: I'm not sure. I'd like to think about this a little more.

HELPER: I get that. You want to make sure what you choose will work for you, and maybe we should look at other ways of getting you over the hump until a bed opens. You want to do residential, and we need to still troubleshoot this waiting period, so you have the best chance of getting your kid back. [Simple reflection, reinforcing change talk] What other ideas do you have? [Open question, partnership]

Planning with Coerced Families

Sometimes, planning may involve reiterating choices within a range of options, including the option not to change. Sometimes, that is the most collaborative stance you can have, especially when the family goal may be mandated by a third party. Autonomy within limits is sometimes the best we can do. The biggest trap I've observed is for frustrated, but well-intentioned, helpers telling the clients that they "have to do something." That violates family members' autonomy. Instead, when planning in MI, helpers generally ask before they inform about options. For example, in the case study we've used in this chapter, the helper asked what the family wanted to do before advising them on what first steps they should take.

Autonomy within limits is sometimes the best we can do.

Planning with Mandated Treatment Plans

In some settings, accreditation or billing standards require certain items to appear on treatment plans. For example, in a substance use treatment center where I worked, it was a requirement to offer all clients an HIV test. This is no doubt a worthwhile requirement. Yet, this could be presented to clients as a "you will have to" or in a collaborative, empathic manner. For example, a helper could say, "One of our funding requirements is to offer all clients an HIV test. I'm wondering what your thoughts are?" One-size-fits-all treatment plans that are autogenerated by technology could either free up clinicians for such MI-style conversations or they could be used in rote fashion with little client input.

Exercise 10.1 demonstrates the connections between focusing, evoking, planning, and the ROARS skills. Try to imagine which of the tasks (focusing, evoking, planning) is furthered with each statement.

EXERCISE 10.1. Focusing, Evoking, or Planning?

Directions: This chapter describes three of the four tasks of MI: focusing, evoking, and planning. In the space to the right, indicate which of these tasks the helper's response is addressing. Note: A response can address more than one task.

Client statement	Helper statement	Task
"I'm not too keen on being here."	"This is hard for you, and yet you came. What would be a good use of this time for you?"	
"We know what we need to do, but we're a bit lost."	"You're both hoping that together we can make a plan that will work for you."	
"I know we should do more things together as a family. It's just hard to find the time."	"It's one more thing to do, and on the other hand, you know you'll all benefit from hanging out more."	
"What do you think we should do?"	"I have a lot of thoughts based on what I've done with prior clients in similar situations. I'm happy to share them with you. But I want to preface this by saying it's important to me that we find something that works for you. So, please feel free to take or leave any of my suggestions."	
"There are so many things going on. It's all too much."	"It's overwhelming. And now your dilemma is figuring out where you want to start."	
"I'm not sure this treatment is the right fit for me."	"You have serious doubts that this will get you where you want to go, and you're also very committed to doing something."	

THOUGHT QUESTIONS: (1) How do you usually know that it is time to plan for change? (2) How much time do you typically spend talking with clients about the reasons they want to change? (3) In what type of situations do you find the most difficulty achieving a focus?

SUMMARY

The four tasks of engaging, focusing, evoking, and planning are a heuristic to remind ourselves to think through timing issues with families. You cannot run (plan) before you walk (engage). And you can engage too long when families are ready to move on. That may be equally frustrating to families. I have called this the superfluous engagement trap. At some point, families want to draw on our expertise and get guidance through change processes. Finally, another key point is that these tasks can overlap, and you can see elements of them even in the same session. Now, let us turn our attention to ending relationships with our families on a positive note, or what I will refer to as motivational sendoffs.

CHAPTER 11

Motivational Sendoffs

> Parting is such sweet sorrow.
> —WILLIAM SHAKESPEARE

Motivation can change at any time, including at the end of helping relationships. Thus, when parting with clients, efforts to build or maintain motivation remain at the forefront of the helper's tasks. In some scenarios, termination involves planful consolidation of commitment to gains made during the helping relationship. There is very little research on these types of endings, with much more focus on when services end abruptly (Norcross et al., 2017).[1] Thus, in this chapter, I demonstrate how we can apply the concept of reinforcing change language in family work with successful terminations. Then, we will turn our attention to applying MI to other types of endings.

Helpers should treat all family interactions as if they were their last. When helping relationships end, family members should leave feeling heard, understood, and in active contemplation of their motivation. This may be motivation for either initiating or sustaining changes. I call this a motivational sendoff. Importantly, we should provide motivational sendoffs to all families we see, regardless of whether they have changed in ways we think are beneficial.

Treat all interactions with a family as if they were your last.

---

[1] I refrain from using the term "dropout," especially in reference to family members. Instead, I use more neutral and person-first terms like "when services end abruptly" or "families who chose to end services." Framing early exits from treatment as "dropouts" is inconsistent with the humanizing spirit of MI and emphasis on family members' autonomy.

This chapter reviews how different motivational sendoffs may look, which hinges on the circumstances under which helping relationships end. For ease of recall, we consider a few such circumstances: planned successful terminations, planned uneasy terminations, uneasy unplanned terminations, and unplanned successful terminations.

CAVEATS

Before describing motivational sendoffs, let me make two caveats. First, these different types of terminations may, in fact, bias the helper's perspective. There is something unsettling when services end before family members implement changes. MI supports the autonomy of family members, which should extend to decisions regarding when to end services. Second, for some types of family work, the concept of termination does not make conceptual sense. For example, in hospital social work, a helper may only have two 15- to 20-minute encounters with family members. Thus, beginnings and endings are one and the same. The concept of termination may apply more to family work with multiple planned sessions.

> Client autonomy extends to deciding when to end services.

PLANNED SUCCESSFUL TERMINATIONS

Planned successful terminations occur when, because of progress, family members and helpers mutually agree that continuing services will lead to diminishing returns. During such terminations, the helper task of consolidating commitment takes center stage. This is achieved through many of the same skills previously described in this book, such as affirmation, reflection, and open questioning. These skills are used to convey empathy and emphasize commitment language.

Example: Termination with Consolidating Commitment

Because previous examples in this book dealt primarily with building motivation in earlier stages of the helping relationship, what follows is an example of what this may look like during termination. The family was on the brink of experiencing a divorce, and one parent suffered from a substance use disorder. In this scenario, a family improved their communication (family-level target behavior), one parent made progress on eliminating their substance use (multilevel target behavior linked to family-level target behavior), and another parent worked on their communication and self-care following the principles of the CRAFT model (Smith & Meyers, 2007).

HELPER: As we've discussed, today I was hoping we could wrap up this experience, celebrate some victories, and look forward. What else should be added to today's agenda? What would make our last session together most helpful to you?

PARENT 1: Well, I want to chat about what we should do if things go south again. I know we're in a better place, but it's still early in my recovery.

PARENT 2: They're doing so much better.

HELPER: It sounds like you're nervous about ending our services. You've all come so far and want to keep that momentum going. Besides celebrating 90 days of sobriety, what other changes should we celebrate in the broader family?

CHILD: I'm not as stressed at home anymore.

HELPER: (*to child*) You're feeling safer because of changes you and your family have made. What have you noticed that is better? What sticks out?

CHILD: We listen to each other, and there is a lot less fighting.

HELPER: (*to child*) So, would you be willing to tell your parents directly about the changes you've seen using your "I statements"? You know the drill (*smiling*).

CHILD: I feel so much better now that you are not fighting. I thought counseling was stupid in the beginning . . . but now I see how much you've worked on getting better. I appreciate that.

HELPER: You've all gotten so well at speaking your mind directly to each other. And you two, what changes have you noticed in your kiddo?

PARENT 1: (*speaking directly to child*) I have seen you snap at us less, and you have really gotten better at being playfully sarcastic but knowing when it goes too far and is hurtful. That helps me because I used to get so stressed out when you did that.

PARENT 2: I couldn't agree more. We both love you so much.

HELPER: You're all in this together and have really improved your communication. So, what are your thoughts on keeping this going as we end our time here?

Parent 1: Well, like we talked about, we'll keep practicing the skills we learned here. And the big thing for me is that, if I have a flare-up with my drug use, I'll go back to treatment or do more online meetings. But, you know . . . once I put drugs in this body . . . that may all go by the wayside.

Helper: (*to Parent 1*) You're really committed to abstinence because for you, once you start, things get unpredictable. So, maybe we should all talk about ideas on how to get back on track if things get unpredictable.

Parent 2: (*to Parent 1*) I wonder if you'd be willing to write and sign a letter to yourself that I hold onto and show you if you go back to using. In the letter, you can include all the reasons you said you didn't want to use and all the changes that happened when you quit. I can keep doing the skills I've been taught, like not arguing when you're high, and trying to arrange non-drug-related fun activities.

Helper: That's so creative. And I like how you phrased that, and how you express your willingness to help. I'm curious, too, how your practice of the CRAFT skills has changed you.

Parent 2: I think I'm less stressed by their behavior. I feel . . . empowered. You know, I can actually see how I'm helping our family change.

Helper: You've worked hard, and it is amazing to see you so committed to continuing to support their sobriety and also take care of yourself.[2]

Clearly, more activities can transpire in final sessions including setting up plans for booster sessions, linking to additional outside resources, or being more thorough about planning for dealing with deterioration. However, in this example, I have chosen to deliberately focus on strategies used in MI to elicit or reinforce change language. Here, in the context of planned successful terminations, reinforcing change language can involve affirmation and reflections. Please recall that these skills can be used at the family or individual level. At the family level, affirmations, open questions, and reflections in the example are addressed to the entire family.

---

[2] I deliberately did not label helper behaviors in this case example so that readers who wish to can practice identifying which skills are which. For a practice activity, and using previous chapters as a guide, consider writing down what skills the helper is using in parentheses after they are used (i.e., family-level affirmation, simple reflection, family-level reflection, etc.).

PLANNED UNEASY TERMINATIONS

Planned uneasy terminations are exactly what they sound like. They are those that occur after some time has elapsed in a helping relationship and there appears to be little movement toward either focusing on or achieving goals. Some families set goals and, when later checking in on progress, don't seem to follow through with mutually agreed-upon homework to do outside of sessions. Or perhaps there has been a ruptured relationship between the helper and family members, and the family has decided to move on to another provider. Other families cannot get past heated interactions, which precludes any focused goal setting. In the family therapy literature, this is often referred to as an *impasse* (Couture, 2006, Heatherington et al., 2005). There are strategies that are used in family work to address impasses, such as sculpting activities (Papp et al., 2013) or observing and altering negative family interactions after reframing them in systemic terms (Diamond & Liddle, 1996). For example, family sculpting, where clinicians ask families to rearrange themselves physically to visually show family relationships and structures, can help resolve impasses. Sometimes, however, family members simply cannot navigate through these difficulties and terminate services.

If strategies to resolve impasses fail, and there are explicit or implicit indications that a family may be considering ending services, some steps can be taken to provide a motivational sendoff. Examples include giving double-sided reflections that stress commitment to change, regardless of the route toward change (e.g., "This wasn't how you were hoping this would go, and yet are still going to look for solutions when we wrap up"), emphasizing autonomy to make decisions about whether to cease services, refocusing on what would be more helpful than the current services offered, or having individual MI sessions with family members whose participation is critical for family work to succeed (see Chapter 9).

Example: Termination with Supporting Autonomy/Looking Forward

In the following example, one partner in couples therapy felt singled out by the helper, in part because their spouse initiated the family therapy process. Thus, they felt the process was stacked against them from the very beginning. In this scenario, two spouses couldn't come to terms on priorities for services. This spouse that ultimately decided to cease services wanted to focus on financial issues and the other spouse on relational issues. Efforts to resolve this impasse failed, and the couple started missing sessions. What follows is a brief call to the partner who is more adamant about ceasing services.

HELPER: I noticed you missed your last couple of sessions and just wanted to check in with you on how things were going. How've you been?

AGGRIEVED PARTNER: So-so. We're talking a little nicer to each other, but I'm just not willing to budge on some things.

HELPER: You're stuck on some things, and yet you're still committed to working things out.

AGGRIEVED PARTNER: Yes, we're not going to see eye to eye on money ever, and to be blunt, I felt like my spouse brought me to you to get you to change me. I feel bad for leaving without saying anything, but you know, it just wasn't for me.

HELPER: This wasn't the right fit for you, and you were worried that I had a strong agenda to side with your partner. Yet, you're still going to keep trying to improve things for you and your family. What are you thinking of trying?

AGGRIEVED PARTNER: I found some money management seminars that we're going to attend together. It may not help with other communication stuff or parenting issues, but she's willing to meet me halfway with some of my concerns about our differences on money. That's the most urgent issue we have. Their shopping is out of control.

HELPER: For you, it makes sense to start there, and you may be willing to revisit other aspects of your relationship once you've made headway on that.

AGGRIEVED PARTNER: Absolutely. If your house is burning down, you don't go to the doctor first. You need a fireman.

HELPER: Great metaphor . . . and thanks for your honesty. It's just not the right time for you to work on other things. I support your approach and wish you well. And you know where to find me if you ever decide that I may be helpful to your family in the future.

AGGRIEVED PARTNER: Thanks, doc. We'll be in touch if we need to.

This brief call shows how a helper can initiate one more short contact to provide a motivational sendoff. This may be beneficial when things do not proceed as we would like in a systemic therapy approach. Many of my colleagues over the years have used the expression "planting seeds" for coping with such unsettling endings. Here, the MI emphasis on autonomy respect co-exists seamlessly with the technique of reinforcing change about other goals (i.e., financial planning). The helper remained steadfastly focused on building motivation for the family member to continue doing something positive for the family, even if they would no longer meet. Perhaps this family will return at a future time.

It would be tempting for helpers to try to convince family members to stay in services if they felt the family had not yet achieved much change. In my field of substance use disorder treatment, there is a longstanding view of holding people in services for a minimum of 90 days. When family members leave treatment earlier than we would have liked them to, it is unsettling. Yet, to practice MI is to acknowledge the many paths to wellness and families' autonomy to choose how to change. Thus, helpers practicing MI should learn to manage negative reactions associated with messy endings. Personal discomfort about whether services were successful or not could inhibit the provision of motivational sendoffs. Failure to manage this discomfort could result in confronting families or engaging in other unhelpful behaviors that run contrary to the practice of MI. For example, attempting to convince a family to persist in a helping relationship they perceive as unhelpful is an autonomy violation. Autonomy respect extends to families' decisions to cease services.

Persuading a family to persist in a helping relationship they perceive as unhelpful is an autonomy violation.

UNPLANNED TERMINATIONS: UNEASY AND SUCCESSFUL

In the previous example, the helper contacted the family member that decided to stop services. However, many times there may be no response from family members. In these situations, helpers are left pondering what became of these families. When there are many unresolved problems or significant ambivalence about change, it can be hard to stay optimistic about family members' outcomes. The best way to provide motivational sendoffs to families with unplanned terminations is simply to stay adherent to MI in all sessions.

Unplanned and Uneasy

In Table 11.1, I've suggested that the best way to provide motivational sendoffs to families that end services involves *ending on empathy*. Perhaps the best way to do this is using an end-of-session summary that clearly demonstrates empathy for the family members present. When routinely practiced, family members' last interactions with helpers were positive.

Example: Termination Ending with Empathy

What follows is an end-of-session summary delivered by a helper to a parent–child dyad at the second session. The teenage child was under court

TABLE 11.1. Motivational Sendoffs

	Planned	Unplanned
Successful	Consolidate commitment	End on empathy
Uneasy	Support autonomy and look forward	End on empathy

supervision for a litany of charges, such as substance use possession, petty theft, and fighting. The parent was at their wit's end, expressing that the child should just straighten up. In the first two sessions, the helper tried to establish an empathic environment and engage both parties into services and frame the youth's problems in family systems. The family did not return for services after this second session.

"So, you've both come to a critical decision point. You've been asked to see me by court services and don't like this. That makes sense because, from what you've said, you both have great problem-solving skills and want to figure things out yourselves. You (*to parent*) have raised two other kids who are doing well and resent that the court asked you to be involved. You value your time so much that you're contemplating whether this is worth the investment. I respect that. It seems like a good way to make decisions. On the other hand, you're both feeling pressure to do something differently. You've both said that it would be amazing for them (*to child*) to be off probation, doing better in school, and on track to be a successful adult. It would lower the number of hassles in both your lives. Today, you shared some thoughts about how to stay out of trouble and are feeling pretty confident you can do it. So, in the coming sessions, I'd like to continue focusing on how to use this time in a way that will be most helpful to you. What else, if anything, would you like to discuss before we end today?"

Some colleagues I've talked to over the years are uncomfortable in situations where families are mandated for services. Some are even more uncomfortable using statements that emphasize autonomy with such families. The logic is that lives are at stake and, if they do not cajole them to remain in treatment, bad things will happen to them. Be that as it may, an alternative viewpoint for not using persuasive or confrontational tactics to retain families is that they may backfire. Families that are reluctant about services may become even more reluctant if they leave services with a bad impression of helpers. As we've discussed before, confrontation and persuasion may trigger sustain talk and keep families stuck. On the other hand, families receiving motivational sendoffs may be more likely to reengage later due to leaving helping relationships with as positive an experience as possible.

Unplanned and Successful: Reason for Optimism?

Ending on empathy is also an excellent strategy for working with families who discuss improvement and abruptly end services. Unlike the previous example, such end-of-session summaries may be more likely to focus on changes that have already happened in the time the helper has seen the family. However, the general principle is the same. End-of-session summaries with families that are doing well provides us with an opportunity to reflect on and affirm their efforts. If they end services abruptly because of rapid progress, such summaries may leave them with positive experiences with helpers.

End on empathy.

The Family Member Who Disappeared

A new client approached me for services after their spouse dissolved their marriage. The client's drinking had increased post-divorce. We met several times, and then they abruptly decided to stop seeing me. They had a strong desire to stop drinking but found services wanting.

From my perspective, they were not in great shape when they stopped services. The client used alcohol heavily and experienced severe depression. To make matters worse, the global COVID-19 pandemic exacerbated their problems. Someone close to them ended their life in the early months of the pandemic.

Throughout our time together, I felt that I did well adhering to MI principles. I never tried to strong arm them into going to support meetings and responded to their ambivalence about change with empathy, autonomy respect, and decent reflective listening that focused on change language.

This family member contacted me about a year after ceasing services. They texted to tell me they were doing well. They had remarried, stopped drinking, and were more physically active. This highly rewarding experience reminded me that I sometimes do a terrible job making prognoses.

THOUGHT QUESTION: What assumptions do you typically make of family members who leave your services with several unresolved issues?

A lot of change can happen in early sessions. And perhaps that is why some families stop coming. The trouble is, unless our former clients contact us after deciding to end services abruptly, we are left with uncertainty about how they fared. Sometimes, however, helpers have rewarding follow-up contact with such families telling their helper that they are doing better. So, as one behavioral therapist told me, helpers may be in a precarious position of having a "slim reinforcement schedule." That is, without feedback loops, we may ruminate or take it personally when families end helping relationships abruptly. At the risk of exuding too much optimism, I encourage readers to humbly consider family members' potential for rapid changes with or without our help, listen carefully to their personal reactions when family members' abruptly end services, and to reflect on opportunities to practice respecting family members' autonomy in such situations. In the box above, I discuss a rewarding experience I had with a family member who ended services prior to achieving goals according to my vision for them.

Exercise 11.1 provides you with an opportunity to practice what you have learned in this chapter. In this exercise, you can practice how to best provide a motivational sendoff to families with each of these four types of terminations from services.

SUMMARY

Humbly acknowledging that there are many pathways to change is difficult for helpers. This may manifest in how helpers approach families at the time of termination. In this chapter, I have advocated for the use of motivational sendoffs, which, among other things, involves emphasizing autonomy, even when it makes the helper uneasy. As termination happens unexpectedly, I also encourage helpers to invest time in ending sessions with summaries that use motivational interviewing skills.

EXERCISE 11.1. Practicing Motivational Sendoffs

Directions: Below are some statements that family members make in the very last session you are having with them. Use the space to think about a response that would help you either consolidate the family's commitment to maintaining changes (planned-successful), support their autonomy and look forward (planned-uneasy), or end on empathy (unplanned-successful and unplanned-uneasy).

Client statement	Type	Helper response
"We simply cannot continue this treatment. We still want to learn how to communicate better but don't see how you can help us. You don't know our family or understand what it's like in our culture. We like you as a person, but I think this is going to have to be our last session."	Planned-uneasy	
"Things are so much better. We are enjoying each other's company more. There is less fighting and a lot less stress. I think the habits we've gotten into, with your help, have really taken hold. We're a little nervous about maintaining this, but we know where to find you if we hit any big bumps in the road."	Planned-successful	
"I am willing to come to these parenting classes. I think that they're really going to help me get the social worker and judge off my back." (Note: Client does not come back for sessions after this statement.)	Unplanned-uneasy	
"Nothing seems to work. We keep trying new therapies, new medications, and it all just seems to end the same."	Unplanned-successful	

THOUGHT QUESTIONS: (1) What do you think will be your biggest challenges with ending sessions on empathy? (2) How do you cope with families that leave treatment before you want them to? (3) What is a good memory you have of a successful family's last session?

PART III

FAMILY-CENTERED MOTIVATIONAL INTERVIEWING RESEARCH

CHAPTER 12

Families Raising and Launching Children

with Alex Lee

> So much is asked of parents, and so little is given.
> —VIRGINIA SATIR

Families face diverse challenges when navigating developmental stages. Research reveals that parent-involved MI effectively improves outcomes among families with children, adolescents, and young adults (Borrelli et al., 2015; Cushing et al., 2014; Ellis et al., 2017; Kao et al., 2023). This chapter assesses existing family-centered MI adaptations for youth from birth through young adulthood.

In this chapter, for each stage of childhood, we provide a brief overview of relevant developmental theories and tasks. Next, we summarize key considerations for implementing family-focused MI in each stage. Finally, we present a practitioner-friendly review of clinical studies demonstrating the efficacy of MI during each stage. We showcase practical MI applications for each phase of family life from early childhood through launching children into adulthood.

Alex Lee is currently a PhD candidate in Social Work at the University of Illinois Urbana–Champaign. He holds a license as a social worker in Taiwan and has extensive experience as a hospital social worker. His research focuses on MI, family-based interventions, and the recovery processes of adolescents from mental health and substance use disorders. His research is dedicated to improving therapeutic strategies and outcomes for youth facing psychological and substance-related challenges.

MI WITH FAMILIES RAISING YOUNG CHILDREN (BIRTH–8 YEARS)

Raising children is simultaneously rewarding and demanding. Parents have a profound influence on their children's development, starting in early childhood. Early childhood, which spans from birth to around 5 years old, is a crucial period for physical, cognitive, and social–emotional development. It lays the foundation for future learning, behavior, and health outcomes. This phase encompasses the infancy (0–2 years), toddlerhood (2–3 years), and preschool ages (3–5/6 years) (Toth & Cicchetti, 1999).[1] Helpers working with families raising young children should be equipped with knowledge about child development. This may facilitate more accurate reflections, avoid blaming parents for their children's problems, and boost motivation for parental tasks that enhance youth development.

Major Developmental Milestones

Young children undergo a series of critical milestones in their gross and fine motor skills (Davis et al., 2011). Cognitively, children are like sponges, absorbing information and making sense of their worlds. According to Piaget (1953), infants build a delicate web of mental frameworks. From understanding basic sensory perceptions to forming more complex ideas about emotions, intentions, beliefs, and problem solving, their cognitive landscapes undergo continuous expansion (Flavell, 1999; Lindenberger, 2001; Piaget & Inhelder, 1969). Interactions with parents, exposure to various stimuli, and engagement in imaginative play contribute significantly to their cognitive development. Social-emotional development in young children encompasses emotional understanding, emotional behavior and feelings, and self-regulation (Denham et al., 2002). Secure attachments with parents allow for emotional connections, while play and group activities refine social abilities (Landry et al., 2003). Because of the importance of attachment in predicting adult outcomes, numerous interventions are designed to prevent maladaptive forms of early infant attachment.

MI Adaptations for Working with Families with Children

Effective interventions for families with children must consider the developmental stage, abilities, and context of each child as well as the family system (Erickson et al., 2005; Toth & Cicchetti, 1999). MI has great potential as a

---

[1] We have included ages 5–8 in this grouping because, after age 8, most studies involve adolescents.

family-based intervention because of its usefulness in engagement, emphasis on empathy, and focus on empowering family members. Parents often feel blamed for their children's problems, and may distrust systems of care. Thus, expressing empathy to parents with young children is critical. Some of their ambivalence about engagement may come from past negative experiences with helping professionals.

> **MI emphasizes empathy and empowering family members.**

Table 12.1 summarizes research on family-based MI focused on families with young children. The findings derived from these evidence-based studies reveals MI is efficacious at reducing some problems experienced by families with young children.

Young Children (Birth-4 Years)

Due to the developmental limitations of younger children under 4, clinical MI studies in this context have predominantly centered around health-related concerns, with parents taking a pivotal role in implementing the family-based interventions.

Oral Hygiene

MI has helped parents monitor and prevent childhood dental decay, a condition with potentially long-term health consequences. Early childhood caries (ECC), or the presence of one or more decayed, missing, or filled teeth before 6 years of age, is a key outcome. Parental involvement and support are significant predictors of positive oral hygiene behavior changes in young children (Dishion et al., 2014; Harrison et al., 2007). So, studies have focused on whether MI can increase parental involvement to improve childhood oral health outcomes.

Study findings are promising. Parent-focused MI led to improved oral hygiene and reduced ECC in infants and toddlers. Weinstein et al. (2004) conducted a randomized trial comparing MI to traditional oral health education for parents. The MI group received one counseling session and six follow-up phone calls, and both groups received educational pamphlets and watched a video. Results showed a lower incidence of new carious lesions in children whose parents received MI compared with education alone. In addition, Faustino-Silva et al. (2019) compared MI and traditional oral health education for parents of toddlers aged 3–4 years. The MI group had less occurrence of ECC compared to those receiving standard education. In summary, two studies show MI is superior to traditional education in promoting early childhood dental health.

TABLE 12.1. Family-Centered MI Studies with Children

Authors	Design	Focus	Objective	Results	Eligibility	Coding
Armstrong et al. (2018)	Randomized	Parents	Children obesity management	Parents receiving MI text messages had better health decision-making process and clinic visit adherence	Parent(s) of children ages 5–12 enrolling in obesity treatments	No
Bean et al. (2019)	Randomized	Parents	Children obesity management	Parents receiving family-centered MI had increased first-time attendance for intervention; no differences were seen in treatment initiation or post follow-up	Parent(s) of children ages 5–11 with body mass index ≥85th percentile	No
Berkel et al. (2021)	Randomized	Parent (FCU)	Children obesity management	Parents involved in the MI program showed an active engagement, attendance, and motivation in interventions compared with the control group	Parent(s) of children ages 5–12 with body mass index ≥85th percentile	No
Blue et al. (2020)	Randomized	Parent	Children oral care	Better child-feeding practice, including improved nighttime bottle habits	Parents(s) of infants <1 year old	No
Davoli et al. (2013) (Italy)	Randomized	Parent	Children obesity management	Improved healthy lifestyle and physical activities, including reduced screen time and reduced eating of unhealthy food	Parent(s) of children ages 4–7 with BMI ≥85th percentile	No
Dawson et al. (2014) (New Zealand)	Randomized	Parent	Children obesity management	Parents were more satisfied with how the information was provided and exhibited higher interest in participating in family-based intervention compared with the control group	Parents(s) of children ages 4–8, recruited from pediatric clinic	No
Dishion et al. (2014)	Randomized	Parent (FCUs)	Improving parenting skills in addressing	Improved parental engagement in treatment and reduced childhood	Parents(s) of children ages 2–5 with	No

Study	Design	Participant	Focus	Outcome	Sample	Behavioral problems
Döring et al. (2016, 2021)	Randomized	Parent	Pediatric obesity prevention	No differences in dietary behaviors in children and mothers; parents showed minimal effect in improving self-efficacy	Parents(s) of children <1 year old	No
Dubose & Dlugonski (2018)	Randomized	Parent	Children physical activity	Improved parent vigorous activity and reduced parent and child sedentary behavior	Parents(s) of children ages 1–5	No
Faustino-Silva et al. (2019) (Brazil)	Randomized	Parent	Children oral care	Better preventive effect against caries, especially among low-income families	Parents(s) of children ages 3–4	No
Harrison et al. (2007)	Randomized	Parent	Early childhood caries prevention	Reduced childhood early caries rates	Parents(s) of children ages 6–18 months	No
Nock & Kazdin (2005)	Randomized	Parent	Childhood behavioral problems prevention	Parents reported a higher motivation in attending treatment programs	Parents(s) of children ages 2–12 with behavioral problems	No
Schwartz et al. (2007)	Randomized	Parent	Pediatric obesity prevention	Reduced snacking, dining-out frequencies, and improved healthy behaviors	Parents(s) of children ages 3–7	No
Shaw et al. (2006)	Randomized	Parent	Early childhood disruptive behaviors prevention	Improved maternal involvement in parenting and reduced childhood disruptive behaviors	Parents(s) of children ages 17–27 months	No
Stormshak et al. (2021)	Randomized	Parent	Enhancing parenting skills during the transition to school	Better parenting skills and reduced caregiver and teacher concerns	Parents(s) of children ages 4–5	No
Weinstein et al. (2004)	Randomized	Parent	Early childhood caries prevention	Better adherence to dental recommendations	Parents(s) of children ages 6–18 months	No

Early Childhood Conduct Problems

To mitigate conduct problems during the transition from preschool to primary school, Shaw and colleagues (2006) implemented the Family Check-Up (FCU), a family-centered intervention incorporating MI. The FCU aimed to sustain maternal involvement and curb worsening conduct issues in children ages 17–27 months. In a 2-year follow-up study, families participating in the FCU showed improved maternal involvement. Their children also displayed less disruptive behaviors like physical aggression.

School-Age Children (4–8 Years)

Pediatric Obesity

MI studies have also addressed pediatric obesity by eliciting parental involvement. Bean et al. (2019) found MI-based interventions effective in lowering obesity risks in children. They employed two MI sessions to guide parents in comprehending healthy eating habits and promoting behaviors that increase physical activity and nutrition. A single session of MI prior to treatment significantly enhanced initial treatment attendance, underscoring the potential for cost and time savings. Armstrong et al. (2018) also examined MI via text messages for parents with children in obesity treatment. While child body mass indices did not notably change, texting substantially reduced attrition in treatment visits. Though more research is needed, these initial studies highlight the promise of family-focused MI techniques to foster parental motivation and engagement in addressing pediatric obesity.

Parenting Skills

Parental ambivalence about improving parenting skills or modeling behaviors, as well as a lack of engagement in programs, may weaken outcomes from empirically supported programs. Thus, two studies have used MI to achieve these ends. Stormshak et al. (2021) also demonstrated the efficacy of the FCU intervention in improving maternal involvement and reducing disruptive behaviors in children transitioning to kindergarten. Helpers delivering this intervention collaborate with parents to build upon existing motivations for enhance parenting skills. Through the utilization of the three-session FCU, which effectively engaged parents and reinforced motivations, the intervention resulted in enhanced child behavioral outcomes.

Additionally, DuBose and Dlugonski (2018) used MI to enhance parent–child motivation to improve physical activity. Coaches helped parents develop healthy strategies and to model motivation to increase their children's physical activity. With eight phone coaching sessions, parents were more likely to engage in vigorous physical activity themselves; their children also displayed less sedentary behaviors. This study demonstrates that family-focused MI can successfully build parental motivation and model positive changes, yielding improved child activity levels.

Finally, MI can increase parents' positive behavior support during early childhood. Dishion et al. (2008) found MI-based interventions effective for improving positive parenting of young children. Practitioners used MI techniques to help parents identify personal strengths and leverage them to enhance parent–child interactions. This highlights the value of MI for engaging parents with young children by drawing out strengths and intrinsic motivation to support their parenting.

> MI can increase parents' positive behavior support during early childhood.

Benefits and Gaps

Early childhood studies on MI show that increasing parental motivation can help improve dental, behavior, and obesity outcomes. For families with young children, helpers are unlikely to use MI directly with very young children, focusing on parents instead. Additional applications of MI could target other early childhood outcomes such as breastfeeding, attachment, or car seat installation, as these targets are known predictors of important child outcomes. Nevertheless, MI shows promise for use in early childhood interventions.

MI WITH FAMILIES WITH ADOLESCENTS (AGES 10–18)

Although there are debates about when adolescence begins and ends, we'll focus here on ages 10–18. This blends the World Health Organizations definition but also acknowledges that age 18 marks the beginning of what some scholars now call emerging adulthood (Arnett, 2000; World Health Organization, 2024).

In early adolescence, individuals traverse significant milestones like puberty, personal identity formation, and building peer relationships (Rice & Dolgin, 2005). MI can play a vital role in helping adolescents navigate evolving roles, responsibilities, decision making, and autonomy (Frey et al., 2011; Miller & Rollnick, 2012; Naar & Suarez, 2021; Rollnick et al., 2016).

This section explores key milestones for families with adolescents and evaluates existing family-centered MI programs tailored to address common challenges. Milestones like increasing peer influence, emerging sexuality, and identity formation accompanied by continued brain development present unique challenges. Family-focused MI offers a collaborative approach to foster the adolescent's burgeoning self-efficacy while eliciting parental wisdom and support during this critical transition.

Major Developmental Milestones

Physical and Cognitive Development

Adolescence involves significant growth in both physical development and cognitive abilities. According to Piaget, adolescents enter the formal operational stage, characterized by abstract thinking, hypothetical reasoning, and considering diverse perspectives (Huitt & Hummel, 2003). Importantly, research in developmental cognitive neuroscience has revealed links between brain maturation and cognitive control. The prefrontal cortex, governing intricate decision making, only fully matures around the mid-20s. This mismatch may help explain adolescents' susceptibility to reward seeking, mood fluctuations, peer influence, substance misuse, and family conflict (Anderson et al., 2002; Steinberg, 2008).

Self-Identity and Autonomy

Adolescent development involves significant identity formation as youth gain greater autonomy from family. Theories such as Erikson's psychosocial model and Marcia's identity status theory emphasize adolescents exploring personal values, beliefs, and aspirations while forging meaningful peer relationships and pursuing independence (Erikson, 1993; Marcia, 1993). This period also entails a transition toward responsibility and independent decision making as adolescents develop an evolving sense of personal agency (Kohlberg & Hersh, 1977). As adolescents begin contemplating their future selves, they frequently experience the challenges of identity confusion (Crocetti, 2017). MI is well suited for adolescents to promote such self-exploration within a nonjudgmental environment (Naar & Suarez, 2021). MI strategies to enhance autonomy may be particularly suited to empowering adolescents.

Parents and Teens

While family influence and support are still critical, it is also essential to recognize adolescents' needs for autonomy and decision making (Whiteman et al., 2011). For instance, increased emotional closeness, support, and interaction with parents during adolescence have been linked to heightened warmth and care (Belsky et al., 2001; Whiteman et al., 2011).

Nevertheless, parents may struggle to adapt to their child's changing appearance and emerging autonomy while providing appropriate supervision and guidance (Lee et al., 2001). Adolescents gain the capacity for logic and introspection but may lack the foresight to make sound choices without parental input. Successfully negotiation on major decisions around dating, academics, and future plans requires perspective taking by both parents and adolescents to understand each other's developmental needs and limitations during this transitional time (Laursen & Collins, 2009).

MI Adaptations for Working with Families with Adolescents

Numerous studies investigated helpers' use MI with adolescents individually, and there is growing interest in family-centered applications. What follows are summaries of family-centered MI studies with adolescents. Additional detail can be found in Table 12.2.

Family Check-Up

As noted above, the FCU is an evidence-based model targeting positive parenting and family well-being (Connell et al., 2016; Dishion & Kavanagh, 2003; Dishion & Stormshak, 2007). The FCU typically consists of two main phases. The initial phase involves establishing family goals, conducting family assessments, and delivering feedback. During the feedback session, professionals employ MI techniques to facilitate constructive dialogue. The second phase focuses on helping families engage in or sustain treatment, guided by the assessment carried out during the FCU. In many research studies, additional multi-level family-centered interventions are integrated (Caruthers et al., 2014; Dishion et al., 2003, 2014; Stormshak et al., 2019; Stormshak et al., 2009, 2021). The strengths-based FCU model assists families in identifying their strengths, addressing concerns, motivating parents, and formulating strategies for positive change.

Extensive clinical evidence underscores the robust impact of the FCU intervention in the past 30 years. For instance, Dishion, Nelson, and Kavanagh (2003) conducted the FCU program with at-risk high school adolescents and their parents, observing a reduction in early substance use and an increase in parental supervision. Moreover, research by Stormshak et al. (2009) indicates that the FCU not only improves student GPA, but also serves as a preventive measure against school absences.

TABLE 12.2. Family-Centered MI studies with Adolescents

Authors	Design	Focus	Objective	Results	Eligibility	Coding
Caruthers et al. (2014)	Randomized	Families (FCU)	Prevention of risky sexual behavior in early adulthood	Family members reported a higher family relationship quality; no differences were seen in risky sexual behavior	Family with adolescents ages 11–12 (6th grade)	No
Chahal et al. (2017)	Randomized	Families	Improving healthy lifestyle for dyslipidemia in adolescents	Lower dietary sugars and screen times	Family with adolescents ages 10–17 with dyslipidemia	No
Connell et al. (2007)	Randomized	Families (FCU)	Prevention of adolescent substance misuse and antisocial behaviors	Teens reported lower rates of substance use, problem behaviors, and arrests by age 18	Family with adolescents ages 11–17	No
Czyz et al. (2019)	Randomized	Families	Adolescent suicide prevention	Better self-efficacy, coping strategies, and parental encouragement	Family with adolescents ages 13–17	No
Dishion et al. (2003)	Randomized	Families (FCU)	Substance misuse prevention	More parental monitoring and less adolescent substance use	Family with adolescents ages 11–12 (6th grade)	No
Fosco et al. (2013)	Randomized	Families (FCU)	Substance misuse prevention	Higher self-regulation and lower rates of antisocial behavior, substance use, and involvement with deviant peers	Family with adolescents ages 11–12 (6th grade)	No

Study	Design	Participants	Focus	Outcomes	Sample	Fidelity
Ghaderi et al. (2018)	Randomized	Families (FCU)	Conduct problems management	Fewer defiant behaviors and conduct problems posttreatment; no differences at 1- and 2-year follow-ups	Family with adolescents ages 10–13 with conduct behaviors	No
MacDonell et al. (2012)	Randomized	Families	Weight management and healthy behaviors	Improved eating behaviors and motivation toward physical activity	Family with adolescents ages 19–17 with body mass index ≥85th percentile	No
Metcalfe et al. (2021)	Randomized	Families (FCU)	Behavioral health management	No difference seen in adolescent rating parental behavior change, but parents self-reported behavioral change (communication, motivation, making progress)	Family with adolescents ages 11–13 with behavioral health problems	No
Pakpour et al. (2015) (Iran)	Randomized	Families	Adolescent obesity management	Better anthropometric, biochemical, psychosocial, and behavioral outcome	Family with adolescents ages 14–18 with body mass index ≥85th percentile	MITI
Sibley et al. (2016)	Randomized	Families	ADHD symptoms management	Adolescents had better OTP skills (organization, time management, and planning), homework completion, parent–teen contracting; parents reported lower stress scores	Family with adolescents ages 11–15 diagnosed with ADHD	No

(continued)

TABLE 12.2. *(continued)*

Authors	Design	Focus	Objective	Results	Eligibility	Coding
Slavet et al. (2005)	Pilot study	Families (FCU)	Substance use prevention	Adolescents had lower substance misuse rates; parents also reported a higher confidence in impacting their adolescents	Family with adolescents ages 15–19	No
Smith et al. (2006)	Randomized	Families (SOFT)	Substance use treatment	Youth randomized to SOFT reduced substance use through 6 months; outcomes were equivalent to an active comparator	Family with adolescents ages 12–18	Yes, reported in Smith et al. (2009)
Spirito et al. (2011)	Randomized	Families	Alcohol use	Youth randomized to individual MI plus FCU had larger reduction in high-volume drinking at 3 and 6 months compared with individual MI only	Family with adolescents ages 13–17	Yes
Stormshak et al. (2009)	Randomized	Families (FCU)	Improving academic performance	Students reported higher GPAs and fewer school absences	Family with adolescents ages 11–17	No
Tucker et al. (2013)	Randomized (quasi-experiment)	Families	Adolescent obesity management	More healthy behaviors and reduced screen time	Family with adolescents ages 11–12 (6th grade) with body mass index ≥85th percentile	No

Research indicates combining the FCU model with other intensive family-centered approaches enhances its efficacy. Integrating the FCU into school-based mental health services improved at-risk students' academic performance (Stormshak et al., 2011). Connell et al. (2016) found the FCU combined with family management treatment reduced adolescent suicide risk into adulthood. Additional evidence supports the FCU's ability to reduce risky behaviors like substance use and risky sexual behaviors when paired with complementary family interventions (Caruthers et al., 2014; Dishon et al., 2003).

Behavioral Health

Incorporating family-centered MI also appears efficacious for adolescents experiencing mental health problems. By employing MI within the family context or blending MI into family-centered treatment, clinicians can achieve improved engagement, communication, treatment adherence, and lasting behavior change among adolescents managing conditions like ADHD, conduct problems, suicidal risk, and other disorders (Adams et al., 2019; Connell et al., 2016; Ghaderi et al., 2018; Sibley et al., 2016).

Obesity and Weight Management

Additionally, clinical evidence supports using MI involving parents when targeting adolescent health issues such as obesity (MacDonell et al., 2012; Tucker et al., 2013) and weight management (Pakpour et al., 2015). For example, Pakpour et al. (2015) conducted a randomized study comparing treatment as usual (TAU), adolescent MI, and family-centered MI for 357 Iranian adolescents with obesity. They found that family-based MI had significantly better outcomes at 12-month follow-up compared with adolescent-only MI.

Substance Use Prevention and Treatment

It is widely recognized that support systems are crucial for both effective prevention and retention in adolescent substance use treatment (Belmontes, 2018). Extensive research affirms the effectiveness of family-centered MI for improving youths' self-regulation of substance use and parents' confidence in monitoring their teens. For instance, Connell et al. (2007) applied the FCU to high-risk adolescents and their parents, specifically targeting risky substance use. Following the intervention, adolescents whose parents participated exhibited less pronounced increases in alcohol, tobacco, and marijuana use, as well as a reduction in problem behaviors between the ages of 11 and 17. They also faced a decreased risk of substance use diagnoses and fewer arrests by the age of 18.

Other family-centered substance use treatments for adolescents include Smith and Hall's (2008) Strengths-Oriented Family Therapy (SOFT) model and Spirito and colleagues' (2011) hospital-based MI study. Smith and colleagues (2006) showed that MI combined with multifamily groups and individual counseling resulted in equivalent substance use outcomes when comparing teens assigned to SOFT or those receiving the Seven Challenges, an active comparison group. Family and individual treatments were provided by the same therapists, and both sets of youth had parental involvement in their initial baseline assessments, in a manner patterned after the FCU. So, the Seven Challenges model was not completely bereft of family involvement, making this comparison somewhat confounded.

Spirito and colleagues (2011) randomized youth admitted to the emergency room with a positive blood alcohol concentration to either individual MI or the FCU. The FCU only produced better outcomes on one alcohol outcome, days of high-volume drinking (i.e., binge drinking). It is unclear why this happened. Some possible explanations are that individual MI is a strong treatment already, family treatments may require longer follow-up periods to show superior effects, or that many families (20%) didn't return for their FCU session. Alternatively, it could just be a statistical problem with showing reduction in a rare variable. That is, the actual change in drinking frequency among adolescents went from about three and a half drinking occasions per month to about two to two and a half drinking occasions per month at follow-ups (Spirito et al., 2011). That does not leave much room for showing major treatment differences.

Benefits and Gaps

Many studies reported positive findings for family-centered MI interventions with adolescents across several change targets. However, further investigation is needed to explore the precise mechanisms by which family-based MI interventions produce positive outcomes. Most studies we reviewed did not include assessments or measurements for the fidelity and quality of MI (17.6%, or 3 out of 17). Future research should consider documenting the adherence to motivational techniques when delivering services. Ongoing clinical research in this area will play a crucial role in enhancing the effectiveness and impact of MI interventions for families in this unique developmental phase.

MI WITH FAMILIES WITH YOUNG ADULTS (AGES 18–29 YEARS)

Young adulthood is a unique, distinct transitional phase bridging adolescence and full adulthood. This period, typically spanning ages 18 to 29, is often referred to as "emerging adulthood" (EA; Arnett, 2000, 2007, Smith, 2017). Emerging adulthood presents a myriad of possibilities, uncertainties, and transformations as "quasi-adults" continue their path toward maturity.[2]

Individually focused MI works well with emerging adults, especially among collegiate populations (Davis et al., 2017). Moreover, extending MI to involve families has shown promise as well. For instance, family motivational intervention (FMI), a form of MI adapted for delivery in a family context, was found to be more successful than standard support methods in addressing cannabis use among young adults with schizophrenia (Smeerdijk et al., 2012). In short, this section explores the developmental milestones of EA, adaptations of family-oriented MI for young adults, and examine the existing clinical evidence.

Major Developmental Milestones
Emerging Adulthood

Arnett (2000, 2007) introduced the concept of EA to capture the shared experiences of individuals between the ages of 18 and 29 in most high-income countries. This phase involves significant progress in self-identity and autonomy, often accompanied by assuming new responsibilities such as managing finances and making decisions about education and career paths. EA is characterized by self-focus, exploration, possibilities, and a sense of being "in-between" (Arnett, 2000).

EA represents a developmental period of heightened vulnerability for engaging in risk-taking behaviors. Similarly to what happens during adolescence, the emerging adult brain undergoes significant changes, particularly in regions responsible for impulse control and decision making. These neurological developments, combined with increased exposure to social contexts that encourage risk taking, may contribute to the prevalence of high-risk behaviors during this phase of life (Arnett, 2000).

The emerging adult brain undergoes significant changes.

---

[2] I say "quasi" because most youth in this age bracket say they feel like adults in some ways, and in other ways they do not feel like adults. This led to Arnett (2000) proposing the concept of emerging adulthood.

Meanwhile, the impulsive system, which responds to rewards and social/emotional influences, develops earlier than the top-down control mechanisms associated with the prefrontal cortex (Casey & Jones, 2010). This imbalance between the impulsive system and the maturation of the frontal lobes may contribute to a propensity for engaging in risky behaviors, such as emerging immediate rewards over long-term goals.

EA and Risky Behaviors

Emerging adults typically exhibit alarmingly elevated rates of substance use disorders, sexually transmitted infections, and other health risks when compared with both older and younger age groups (Johnston et al., 2015; Stone et al., 2012). Importantly, these surges in risk-taking behaviors are not exclusive to college students, highlighting the presence of broader developmental vulnerabilities during this life stage, rather than being solely attributed to campus-related factors (White et al., 2006). The behavior of emerging adults is significantly influenced by the social environment. Peer influences, societal expectations, and cultural norms can shape the adoption of risk-taking behaviors (Arnett, 2007). As young adults strive for autonomy and independence, they become more susceptible to peer pressure and societal norms, which may lead them to engage in risky activities (Stone et al., 2012).

Despite the disproportionately high prevalence of risky behaviors and their associated negative consequences, research indicates that only approximately 5% of emerging adults with substance use disorders receive specialized treatment (Pedrelli et al., 2015). Given this striking disparity between the need for treatment and actual engagement, there is a compelling case for implementing evidence-based interventions or preventive measures tailored to the specific needs of emerging adults.

Shifting of Family Roles

As families navigate the transition into young adulthood, they encounter significant changes in roles and responsibilities. Parents shift from authoritative figures to advisors, while siblings develop relationships as peers rather than as children (Fingerman et al., 2012). As described in the EA theory, this phase marks a crucial stage of self-discovery. Typically, individuals in this phase forge their own distinct social identities by exploring personal values and beliefs and forming relationships outside the family (Arnett 2007; Arnett et al., 2014).

> A crucial state of self-discovery.

Despite this growing independence, Arnett (2000) emphasizes the continued influence and reliance on parents during this period. Additional studies have highlighted the impact of family involvement in mitigating peer influence on substance use and risky behaviors among young adults (Abar & Turrisi, 2008; Wood et al., 2004). As an example, Walls et al. (2009) found that parental permissiveness significantly affects emerging adults' drinking habits and consequences. Furthermore, parents may be reluctant to pressure their young adult children to change their substance use, which is associated with drops in interpersonal motivation to change among emerging adults in treatment (Smith et al., 2010).

Supporting Autonomy and Self-Determination

As suggested by Naar and Suarez (2021), MI is well suited to young adults because of their needs for autonomy. MI provides a mechanism for emerging adults to openly explore internal experiences, values, and motivations related to change (Miller & Rollnick, 2012). Practitioners should foster a nonjudgmental environment for emerging adults to express thoughts/feelings, gain self-insight, and clarify change motivations. MI allows emerging adults to vocalize their desire for independence while eliciting parents' support. This autonomy-supportive approach can smooth the transition to adulthood within the family system.

Clarifying Goals and Values

Young adults tend to be future-oriented, often seeking to establish life goals and a sense of purpose (Arnett, 2015). MI can help align future aspirations with the young person's core values and intrinsic motivations for sustainable change. Practitioners can utilize open questions to explore the dreams and goals of emerging adults in various aspects of their lives, such as careers, relationships, and personal growth. By eliciting their deeper motivations and values, MI helps young individuals bridge the gap between their desired life directions and what truly matters to them.

Parent-Child Relationships

While seeking independence, emerging adults often still depend on their parents emotionally, financially, and mentally (Agliata & Renk, 2008; Aquilino, 2006). Family-centered MI can aid emerging adults in discovering purpose and taking value-aligned steps toward goals. Collaborating with parents provides insights on translating aspirations into actionable plans. With empathy and evocation, MI empowers emerging adults to chart an adulthood path resonating with their values while benefiting from family support. MI fosters enduring personal growth during this transition by aligning goals with motivations.

MI Adaptations for Working with Families with Young Adults

Table 12.3 summarizes family-centered MI research with young adults. What follows are detailed summaries of these studies.

Young Adult Family Check-Up

The Young Adult Family Check-Up (YA-FCU) is designed to promote family engagement and has a track record of reducing problems among young adults through a strengths-based feedback approach following a comprehensive assessment (Dishion & Stormshak, 2007). A central focus of the YA-FCU is to enhance protective factors in parent–child relationships, emphasizing effective communication and nurturing healthy autonomy in emerging adults. This intervention is unique in its use of assessment-driven feedback, employing a collaborative and motivation-enhancing approach that centers on the family system's impact on the motivation and capacity for change in young adults (Stormshak et al., 2019). Moreover, it identifies strategies to support young adults in developing adaptive behaviors aligned with their goals and positive outcomes as they transition to adulthood.

DeVargas and Stormshak (2020) conducted a randomized study examining the outcomes of the YA-FCU on emerging adults' health behaviors. Results demonstrated that higher therapist fidelity to MI principles related to more client change talk during sessions. Additionally, Stormshak et al. (2019) initially conducted a study in which families were randomly assigned to receive the FCU or school as usual during the middle school years. Ten years later, they were offered the YA-FCU, which was adapted for families of emerging adults. The results revealed that the more hours that youth and families were engaged in the YA-FCU, the greater the reductions in young adult risk behavior relative to those who did not engage or engaged very little in the intervention.

Substance Misuse

Research indicates that family-based MI can positively impact substance use in emerging adults. Studies show familial relationships moderate peer

TABLE 12.3. Family-Centered MI studies with Young Adults

Authors	Design	Focus	Objective	Eligibility	Results	Coding
Smeerdijk et al. (2015)	Randomized	Families	Reducing cannabis use and parental stress among families with young adults with schizophrenia	Family with young adults ages 16–35 with schizophrenia and co-occurring cannabis use disorder	Young adults had decreased cannabis use and craving; parents reported less parenting distress and sense of burden	MITI
Stormshak et al. (2019)	Randomized	Families (YAFCU)	Preventing risky behaviors among young adults	Family with young adults ages 20–21	Reduced risky behaviors, such as substance use and high-risk sexual behaviors	No
Turrisi et al. (2009)	Randomized	Families	Preventing substance use among young adults	Family with incoming college students ages 18–21	Lower alcohol consumption, high-risk drinking, and consequences at 10-month follow-up	MITI
Wood et al. (2010)	Randomized	Families	Alcohol misuse prevention among incoming college students	Family with incoming college students ages 18–20	Lower onset of consequences	No
Woodin et al. (2012) (Canada)	Randomized	Couples	Reducing partner aggression among young couples	Couples ages 18–20 with at least one incident of intimate partner violence	Reduced physical aggression behaviors	MITI

pressure's influence on college student drinking (Turrisi et al., 2000; Wood et al., 2004).

Wood et al. (2010) examined combining individual brief motivational intervention (BMI) using MI principles with parent-based intervention (PBI) focused on motivating parents. Students receiving both BMI and PBI showed lower alcohol-related consequences versus BMI alone or no intervention. This suggests engaging emerging adults and parents together enhances outcomes compared to student-only MI for substance use. Additionally, Turrisi et al. (2009) found BMI combined with PBI reduced drinking and consequences more than either alone for high-risk college students. For this population, integrating individual and family MI had a greater impact.

Overall, these findings indicate that involving families through MI, in conjunction with individual interventions, can strengthen outcomes for emerging adults struggling with substance use. Engaging both the young person and their family unit appears to be a promising approach warranting further research.

Intimate Relationships

A key developmental task for emerging adults is forming close, intimate relationships (Arnett 2000). However, violence can emerge in young adult couples as intimacy deepens. Woodin et al. (2012) examined using MI to reduce aggression in college-age couples. In a randomized study of 50 couples, therapists conducted a 2-hour motivational assessment and feedback session with each couple, with follow-ups over 9 months. Results showed higher therapist fidelity to MI principles, measured by the Motivational Interviewing Treatment Integrity (MITI) codes (Moyers et al., 2016), was associated with reduced aggression in both partners. This study concluded that MI is applicable to addressing intimate partner violence, and therapists who more closely adhere to the spirit of MI might obtain better outcomes in terms of behavior change.

Benefits and Gaps

Family-centered MI holds promise in supporting young adults during their transitional phase. However, there are notable limitations to consider. First, research on family-centered MI with young adults remains relatively limited, warranting further investigation to fully comprehend its efficacy and potential variations across different family dynamics and cultural considerations. Additionally, striking the right balance between autonomy and family involvement can be a complex endeavor, as the needs of emerging adults vary widely. Finally, young adults and their families may not live together. Thus, family work with young adults may require virtually delivered sessions.

SUMMARY

This chapter aims to illustrate the adaptability of MI for use with families with children, adolescents, and emerging adults. Clinical trials have provided evidence supporting the efficacy of family-centered MI. It is important to acknowledge that, despite our review of over a hundred clinical studies of family-centered MI, it is unclear if family-centered MI would achieve superior outcomes relative to individually delivered MI. We reiterate that, in many cases, there is limited information about the quality of the delivery of MI. The absence of this critical information makes it challenging to draw definitive conclusions about the specific impact of MI in family settings. Thus, future work should integrate tools such as MITI codes or the MISC to ensure consistency across sessions and facilitate comparisons of outcomes across various studies (Moyers et al., 2016). Nevertheless, because of these findings, we encourage research on MI with families whose children have yet to launch into fully established adulthood.

CHAPTER 13

Families with Established and Older Adults

> Oh, the worst of all tragedies is not to die young,
> but to live until I am seventy-five and yet not ever
> truly to have lived.
> —Martin Luther King Jr.

In modernity, the traditional markers of adulthood have lost a modicum of meaning. Just as the elongation of adolescence by market forces birthed the concept of emerging adulthood (Arnett, 2000), technological and medical advances have also changed the nature of older adulthood. Aging adults will live longer, have access to technologies allowing new forms of social connection, and face new choices. Helping professionals will have increased opportunities working with older adults and their families.

MI is well suited to respect the autonomy and experience of established and older adults. With such rich life experience forged through longevity, helpers may have much to evoke. Older adults have likely experienced successful change efforts at some point in their lives. So, MI appears well suited for use in partnering with older adults to co-create solutions to their current problems.

Tap the experience of established and older adults.

The renowned 19th-century philosopher Søren Kierkegaard wrote that anxiety is an unanticipated byproduct of freedom (Kierkegaard, 2014). And there are now a dizzying number of paths adults may traverse in older adulthood. The forces of globalization and technology give modern people a wide array of choices. Because there are so many paths, we must be prepared for established and older adults who are experiencing ambivalence about these phases of their lives. In the box below, I share my family experiences, upcoming midlife choices, and some associated ambivalence about these decisions.

As experiences vary so widely, we should not rigidly adhere to assumptions about established and older adults. Fortunately, when one practices MI well and with an uncluttered mind, we listen carefully and understand nuances in each older adult's path (Miller & Rollnick, 2023). Knowledge of lifespan development, however, need not be clutter that prevents the use of accurate reflective listening. To the contrary,

Find out about normative developmental tasks in adulthood.

My Midlife Experiences and Ambivalences

As I write this, I am entering my 50th year of life. I have one child finishing college and one finishing high school. Guiding them into adulthood, and seeing who they are becoming, presents great joys and challenges. Furthermore, they cope with some painful health challenges that reverberate through the family. My mother, stepfather, and mother-in-law are in their 70s and 80s. One needs intensive care. This requires my spouse and me to make a 6-hour round trip drive once a month for visits. It is critically important to do, and I wouldn't trade this for anything, yet it is physically and emotionally draining.

I have been at the same job for 16 years. At 20 years, some of my retirement benefits kick in. Choices lie ahead. The timing of my retirement is one. Also, potential opportunities I could pursue in research, clinical, or administrative roles beckon decisions. I ruminate on where my skillset is most needed to contribute to this world. (I think self-reflective social workers are supposed to do that.) I wonder if I'll live in the same city 5 or 10 years from now. Of course, the timing of these decisions is clearly impacted by my family members. I genuinely see multiple paths I could take. The role my privilege plays in these choices is not lost on me.

Because my father passed away in March 2019, and the global COVID 19 pandemic followed that, I feel growing urgency to make decisions. My spouse and I know our genetic risks for potentially upcoming health problems. In many ways, we are ambivalent about what we want to do with the rest of our lives.

THOUGHT QUESTIONS: (1) How may ambivalence look for middle-aged adults of different cultural or socioeconomic backgrounds from mine? (2) In what ways are my midlife experiences like those described in family life cycle perspectives?

knowledge about normative developmental tasks can aid in producing excellent guesses about what family members are communicating. Proficient MI with older adults may be more impactful when helpers simultaneously understand general concepts about aging while listening for and empathizing with family members' diverse experiences. The freedom to age makes assumption-free listening critical when practicing with older adults.

Whereas the previous chapter provided a practitioner-friendly review of MI work with younger families, the focus here is on families with established and older adults. I realize that categorizing families as younger or older is a daunting task, as their intergenerational nature often precludes such clear divisions. Nevertheless, I follow the heuristic of the family life cycle framework presented in Chapter 6. I review all family-centered adaptations of MI that I could locate for established and older adults, note gaps in the research, and make recommendations for the integration of family members in MI practice with older adults.

ESTABLISHED ADULTS (AGES 30–50)

Established adulthood refers roughly to the period of life between the 30s and 50s (Mehta et al., 2020). Notwithstanding myriad life course variations, it is typically when people are busy caring for children and taking care of their elders. These competing, and often stressful, demands can overwhelm established adults' coping resources.

Most work reviewed in Chapter 12 involved parenting interventions using MI with established adults who were caring for a younger child. Here, we summarize nonparenting studies with established adults (see Table 13.1). The main foci of these studies were relationship enhancement and sexual wellness, family-centered care for diabetes and coronary care, and substance use treatment.

Relationship Enhancement and Sexual Wellness

Marriage Checkup

The Marriage Checkup (MC) is a well-researched model that integrates MI into family therapy for adult populations. It was developed as a preventative intervention for at-risk or distressed couples. In the first study on the MC, a preexperimental trial, the authors found global distress was significantly reduced among both partners in heterosexual couples (Cordova et al., 2001). Subsequent studies also found positive effects of this intervention in randomized designs (Cordova et al., 2014; Trillingsgaard et al., 2016). In addition to improving relationship outcomes, one trial found couples receiving the MC had reduced depression symptoms (Gray et al., 2020).

The MC is delivered as a two-session intervention, where the first session involves assessment and the second session involves feedback delivered in a style consistent with MI. Unlike other models of MI that use a similar format, no process coding of MI (i.e., MI adherence measure) was used in any of these studies. Thus, it is unclear to what extent the outcomes in these studies may be driven by the technical processes of MI (i.e., generating change talk). Additional research on whether these MI-specific processes operate as mechanisms of change would be a welcome addition to the literature on this efficacious intervention.

MI for Sexual Wellness

Unlike other couples counseling research, the work of Starks and colleagues (2022a) extensively measured the implementation of MI. Specifically, their couples-focused work centers on substance use and sexual risk behaviors among sexual minority male couples. Relative to a control group, partners in such couples had no significant differences in substance use. However, when they focused on partners with high baseline substance use, they found more promising effects. Furthermore, condomless anal sex was also reduced among participants receiving this MI-infused couples counseling (Starks et al., 2022b). A full description of the clinical model is available elsewhere (Starks, 2022).

Another study investigated the use of couples-focused MI for adopting the use of long-acting reversable contraception (LARC) among Rwandan couples. Delivered as implants, these LARCs are known to reduce the risk of pregnancy and perinatal HIV transmissions (Mukamuyango et al., 2020). MI was delivered in individual sessions to both members of couples. After receiving MI, about a third (34%) of couples who were initially hesitant to use a LARC adopted one.

Diabetes and Coronary Care

A series of studies from the same research lab included family-centered MI in their work with persons from the Marshall Islands with type 2 diabetes (Felix et al., 2019, 2020, McElfish et al., 2019). Family members attended groups where MI was used. This study found evidence for improvements in glucose monitoring and primary care visits (Felix et al., 2019) and lower HbA1C 12 months following the treatment (McElfish et al. 2019). This

TABLE 13.1. Family-Centered MI studies with Established Adults

Authors	Design	Focus	Objective	Results	Eligibility	Coding
Bortolon et al. (2017)	Randomized	Family member	Decreasing codependent behaviors	Family members of person with substance use disorder who completed treatment were twice as likely to reduce codependent behaviors	Family members calling a toll-free number for information on helping loved one with substance use disorder	No
Cordova et al. (2001)	Pre-experimental; nonequivalent comparison group	Couples	Reducing distress and increase relationship satisfaction	Couples receiving the MC had increased marital satisfaction at 1-month follow-up; distress was lower than a community sample not receiving services	Cohabitating married couples seeking help at university clinic	No
Cordova et al. (2014)	Randomized	Couples	Improving intimacy, relational acceptance, and marital satisfaction	Relative to controls, couples had increased intimacy, relational acceptance, and marital satisfaction	Community sample of cohabitating married couples	No
Duncan et al. (2016)	Randomized	Families	Reducing obesity and cardiovascular risks	Total cholesterol, fast-food consumption, and body mass index were all lower at 12 months	Ages 35–65 with cardiovascular risk and high body mass index	No
Felix et al. (2019)	Randomized	Families	Diabetes management	Greater glucose monitoring and physician visits	Participants ages 18+ and at least one additional family member	No
Felix et al. (2020)	Within-condition analysis	Families	Diabetes management	No differences in health outcomes between family members attending one or more versus no sessions	Analysis of family members supporting participant meeting eligibility criteria	No

Study	Design	Sample	Outcome	Results	Sample Description	Fidelity Measure
Gray et al. (2020)	Randomized	Couples	Depression	Reduced depression symptoms	Couples residing in New England	No
McElfish et al. (2019)	Randomized	Families	Diabetes management	Lower HbA1C through 12 months relative to control group	Participants ages 18+ and at least one additional family member	No
Morris et al. (2018)	Randomized	Separated couples	Parenting agreements	More agreements among couples in MI-based mediation	Separated couples making parenting arrangements	MITI
Mukamuyango et al. (2020)	Pre-experimental	Couples	Promoting use of LARC	34% of couples chose to use a LARC after MI session	Couples who wanted to delay pregnancy for at least 2 years but had not done so at 1-month follow-up	No
Project MATCH Research Group (1998)	Randomized	Couples	Increasing percent days abstinent and reduce heavy drinking days	MI outcomes were equivalent to active comparison groups; MI was better than other treatments for persons with high trait anger	One target client with an alcohol use disorder and their CSO	MISO
Starks et al. (2022)	Randomized	Couples	Reducing substance use and condomless anal sex (CAS)	No significant differences in overall analyses; significant reductions in substance use and CAS among couples with high baseline frequencies	Sexual-minority male couples where at least one member used substances and at least one had CAS outside the relationship	MITI
Trillingsgaard et al. (2016)	Randomized	Couples	Increasing couple satisfaction, safety, and responsiveness and attentiveness	MC outcomes were better on all four outcomes at 54-week follow-up	Danish couples recruited in the community for treatment at a private practice	No

group also studied the impact of the treatment on family members who attended to support a targeted individual with type 2 diabetes. Unfortunately, there was no evidence for improvements in their health indicators, and the authors specifically recommended that methods be studied to improve family member engagement. Increasing the engagement of family members in such treatments would permit stronger research on whether the benefits of family-centered interventions extend beyond the target client.

Family-centered interventions for established adults at risk for experiencing a coronary event have also integrated family members. Duncan and colleagues (2016) involved family members in home visits as part of a multicomponent intervention. Their intervention was successful in reducing body mass index, fast food consumption, and total cholesterol at 12 months (Duncan et al., 2016).

Substance Use Treatment

William Miller, the lead developer of MI, dedicated his career to working with people with alcohol use problems. Thus, it is no surprise that some work with established adult families stemmed from large alcohol use disorder treatment trials. Below, I give a brief overview of this work. These studies on alcohol treatments included identified patients with alcohol use disorders and integrated one concerned significant other to support their change efforts.

Project MATCH

The seminal study on alcohol use disorder treatment for adults included one motivational enhancement therapy (MET) condition, where adults could bring a concerned significant other (CSO) to their sessions. Because it was optional, most likely to respect diverse family constellations and client autonomy, approximately 34.7% of study participants included a CSO (Manuel et al., 2012). They included romantic partners (81.5%), parents (11.1%), friends (3.7%), and children. This study included CSOs to raise their awareness about the identified patient's drinking and treatment goals, activate social support, and problem-solve barriers to achieving goals.

In this study, MET was as efficacious as the other treatments in Project MATCH, including cognitive-behavioral (CBT) and twelve-step facilitation (TSF) therapies. Furthermore, there was no matching effect. That is, the logic of the study design was that, if individuals with low motivation received MET (via random assignment), they would do better than similar clients with lower motivation receiving CBT or TSF (Longabaugh & Wirtz,

2001). This is because MI is specifically designed to increase motivation. So, it would make sense for individuals with low motivation to have better alcohol outcomes if they received MET. Ultimately, however, individuals with lower motivation who received MET did not have better outcomes. However, those who had elevated anger had better outcomes in MET. Additionally, individuals with poorer social support had better outcomes in TSF (Project MATCH Research Group, 1998).

TSF treatment worked better for people without stable social support, perhaps allowing people to choose new "selected," rather than biological, family members. TSF was designed to promote social support seeking through twelve step participation. Yet, family participation was optional in the MET treatment, since the study was designed to test the impact of changes in motivation, not the impact of social support. Perhaps this was also due to MI's emphasis on client autonomy, in this case, autonomy to choose whether to bring a CSO. One question raised by this finding of low attendance is whether additional efforts are needed to boost family member inclusion in situations where clients have an available CSO.

COMBINE

An additional large multisite study attempted to evaluate the synergistic effects of combined behavioral and pharmacological treatments for established adults with alcohol use disorders (Anton et al., 2006). Notably, significant other attendance in the combined intervention improved outcomes. However, only 26.9% of identified patients in the study brought CSOs (Hunter-Reel et al., 2012). These individuals who brought CSOs to at least one session had better outcomes than those who did not. This speaks to the importance of engaging individuals reluctant to include their family members in treatment.

Other Substance-Related Studies

Barbara McCrady and colleagues have long studied whether strengthening couples' relationships can improve alcohol treatment outcomes (McCrady et al., 2016). In alcohol-focused behavioral couples therapy (ABCT), helpers address relational issues and alcohol use disorders simultaneously. It is not a treatment specifically designed to increase change talk, like MI, so I did not include it in Table 13.1 as a family-centered MI study. However, some studies have researched whether change talk may be operating as a mechanism of change in ABCT (Fokas et al., 2020; McCrady et al., 2019). For a full summary of these studies refer to Chapter 8.

One additional family-centered study tested whether an adaptation of MI could help family members reduce codependent behaviors in support of a family member with a substance use problem (Bortolon et al., 2017). This Brazilian study found a reduction in codependent behaviors among family members receiving MI relative to those in the control group.

ADULTS IN THEIR 50s AND BEYOND

MI is efficacious with older adults. Numerous studies show its benefits in adult protection services (MacNeil et al., 2023), health promotion (Tellez et al, 2019; Tse et al., 2013), disease management and medication adherence (Kang & Gu, 2015; Moral et al., 2015; Shertz et al., 2019), and communicating with pharmacists about medications (Martin et al., 2016). In short, MI is increasingly used in health care contexts frequented by older adults.

However, after an exhaustive search,[1] I found limited work on family-based adaptations of MI where a significant portion of the sample were senior citizens. The one exception was a study by Miklavcic and colleagues (2020), who invited caregivers to sessions with seniors living with type 2 diabetes. In this randomized study, participants did not significantly improve their physical functioning at a 6-month follow-up. No data on family attendance at in-home sessions were reported. I encourage researchers and clinicians working with other adults to consider whether engaging supportive family members with MI may increase such attendance.

In another study, family members participated in an intervention targeting seniors 65 years of age and older following coronary bypass surgery. However, family members were not included in MI sessions, but rather attended psychoeducational sessions only (Lin et al., 2017). Medication adherence and lipid profiles were better in the intervention group. I recommend the use of family-centered MI in psychoeducational groups whenever possible. Such adaptations could possibly circumvent time-constraint pressures in many care settings.

Use family-centered MI in psychoeducational groups.

Considering the scarcity of family-centered MI work with seniors, I review some developmental considerations pertaining to older adults. Then, I comment on practice areas where MI has been used with seniors in individual session format, giving recommendations on areas where families might be integrated.

---

[1] I searched multiple databases and screened over 1,000 abstracts for any studies on family-based MI outcome studies.

Developmental Considerations

For older adults, several normative considerations bear mentioning. First, depending on their cognitive capacities, older adults may need MI delivered at a slow pace or with the use of strategies to enhance retention of concepts. MI may not be appropriate for individuals with advanced dementia (Abughosh et al., 2017). Additionally, remember that older adults may be using multiple medications, have interconnected medical problems, and possibly be experiencing grief or loss (Sedarevic & Lemke, 2013). Physical abilities decline. Furthermore, elders face complicated emotions about their own mortality. Maintaining social connections in older adulthood is a known predictor of quality of life and health outcomes (O'Rourke et al., 2018). It is no surprise then, that many studies use MI to address advance care planning, physical activity, and social connection.

Opportunities for Family Integration

Advanced Care Planning

Only 46% of seniors legally document their medical preferences for end-of-life care (Perumalswami et al., 2021). In the absence of advance care plans, caregivers and other family members may experience substantial stress over medical, placement, and funeral decisions, guessing at their elder's preferences (Fried, 2022). As care planning is a decision about which many seniors may experience ambivalence, MI may be appropriate.

Fried and their colleagues (2021) found that a personalized feedback intervention increased completion of four advanced care planning activities, including communicating with a trusted person about the tension between quality and quantity of life, assignment of a health care agent, having a living will, and having documentation in their medical records. Seniors completed a brief assessment and then received printed and tailored feedback based on each of their readiness to make changes. In intervention sites, 14% of patients completed all these activities, versus 8.2% in usual care sites. The most common advanced planning activity (65%) was speaking with a trusted person about balancing quality and quantity of life in decision making, which, for seniors, likely involved family members.

Another study on advanced care planning found evidence for increased documentation of decisions but lower readiness to speak to family members about their decisions (Nedjat-Haiem et al., 2019). Specifically, seniors receiving MI had significantly lower readiness to talk with family members about advance care planning decisions versus those in a control group. One possible explanation for this is that their clinical protocol involved discussing seniors' barriers to talking with their family members about care planning. Thus, they may have elicited sustain talk in their protocol, which could explain their increased ambivalence about family involvement at posttest. This underscores the need for careful monitoring of treatment adherence. No adherence measures were reported in this study.

Although Fried and colleagues' (2021) study did not involve family members, end-of-life care clearly involves them. Additional possibilities exist for integrating family members into advanced care planning. For example, expanding the settings in which this work is done could be fruitful. Notoriously fast-paced primary care clinics can only accommodate the briefest (a.k.a. scalable) interventions. However, congregate care settings may be able to implement multiple family groups or single conjoint sessions with families of residents. Also, future adaptations of MI could involve addressing caregiver ambivalence to carry out seniors' wishes. Although most seniors in Fried et al.'s (2021) study talked with a trusted person about quality of life, only one in three completed a living will. Thus, execution of seniors' end of life intentions often hinges on their providers and family members.

Adaptations of MI could involve single or multiple caregivers such as romantic partners or adult children, respectively. Examples could include discussions with a senior's romantic partner about how upcoming medical decisions reflect their and the patient's desires. Sometimes, these may be in conflict, as in the case of a romantic partner who disagrees with a patient's desire to cease life-saving measures. Additionally, adult children may have disagreements about how to proceed with their elder parent's care. Decisions could include whether to proceed with a surgery, which type of care setting is appropriate (e.g., in-home or institutional), or whether their parent should remain on preventative medications in an advanced state of dementia. These represent excellent opportunities for empathic listening with distressed family members. However, for both legal and ethical reasons, extreme caution must be exercised regarding generating change talk with these types of decisions. The concept of equipoise likely applies in many end-of-life discussions using MI.

Involve caregivers, such as romantic partners or adult children.

Exercise and Physical Mobility

Declines in physical activity and mobility occur late in life. Some adaptations of MI have addressed these problems but have primarily targeted only seniors (de Vries et al., 2016; Larsen et al., 2021; Tuvemo Johnson et al., 2021). In some studies, elders are encouraged to identify support people to assist their efforts. In some situations, family members have been responsible for helping with physical activity but were not directly targeted by interventions (de Vries et al., 2016).

It is unclear to what extent working through caregiver ambivalence with MI would result in increased family assistance with elders' physical activities. Lengthy sessions focused on eliciting caregiver change talk may not be necessary. However, caregivers are clearly present during some physical activity interventions delivered to elders. Thus, it is possible that brief scalable motivational interventions could target their willingness to help. This could be as simple as delivering brief advice to caregivers after asking them questions on their motivation (e.g., ability, willingness, importance) to help with their elderly family member's exercise efforts.

PRACTICE AND RESEARCH RECOMMENDATIONS

There is a beginning evidence-base for using family-centered adaptations of MI with established and older adults. Addressing four key areas will further enhance our understanding of family-centered MI during these parts of the life cycle. First, even among studies that attempted to integrate family members in interventions, their involvement in interventions appears low. Second, as seen in Table 13.1, few researchers report fidelity measures for their implementation of MI. Third, studies on older adults are largely absent. Finally, outside of couples counseling, family member outcomes are rarely considered.

Family Engagement Varies

One of the key challenges in implementing family-centered MI is promoting the attendance of family members, which is as low as 27%. I interpret this as indicating a need to engage both target clients and family members with MI to increase session attendance. No study reviewed and mentioned here appeared to use MI in this way. In fact, one caveat about this review is that there was often limited information about whether family members actually received MI or whether involvement was only limited to other activities.

What is clear is that when family members participate in multicomponent interventions for established adults that use MI, their treatment outcomes are generally better than control groups. Thus, my hope is that the clinical methods articulated in earlier chapters can be used to engage and retain family members in these interventions.

MI Fidelity

Outside of a few studies, there appears to be limited process coding. Although family therapy research has a long tradition of process coding, these studies are largely not implementations of systemic family therapies. Instead, many are multicomponent family-centered health interventions. They largely did not use either Motivational Interviewing Treatment Integrity (MITI) or Motivational Interviewing Skills Code (MISC) instruments.

The absence of process coding makes it impossible to determine whether MI was delivered as intended in these family-centered studies. Also, it precludes studying whether the ROARS skills or evocation of change talk, presented in earlier chapters, occurs when there is a larger family presence in the room. To determine whether outcomes in family-centered MI treatments are attributable to increases in change talk, such work is encouraged.

Limited Work with Older Adults

Family-centered adaptations of MI appear lacking for older adults. I located only two studies that seemingly integrated family members into services designed to treat heart health and type 2 diabetes. This represents a missed opportunity for implementing family-centered MI. As noted earlier, many studies try to activate social support, and MI can be used for that task when there is ambivalence about doing so.

Beyond Target Client Outcomes

An interesting question is whether people participating in a support role in another person's treatment also experience positive changes. Indeed, in my work with young adults, I've seen supportive friends make positive changes in their substance use. This occurred even though their substance use was not directly targeted by the intervention (Smith et al., 2016). Here, in the context of family-centered MI treatments for established and older adults, only one trial considered this possibility.

Could family-centered MI have positive effects on both elder outcomes and caregiver stress? This highly plausible possibility remains to be tested.

SUMMARY

This chapter reviewed all available family-centered MI studies targeting established and older adults. There were more studies with the former group than the latter. Common foci were couples' relationship functioning, sexual wellness, substance use, diabetes, and coronary care. Four clear recommendations can be made from this work including the need to (1) increase family engagement, (2) use process measures to document the quality of MI and permit study of mechanisms of change, (3) do more family-centered MI work with elders, and (4) broaden the tested outcomes to include those that may be experienced by supportive family members who participate in programs with an identified patient.

APPENDIX

Select Resources for Integrating Motivational Interviewing in Family Work

Here, I highlight a number of resources that may be useful to you for mastering MI. You may obtain some resources free of charge, with others available for purchase. For each resource, I provide a brief description, some suggestions on how the resource can be used for training and learning, and where it may be accessed. As well, links to the respective organizations providing these resources are given at *www.guilford.com/smith10-materials*.

THERAPEUTIC PROCESS INSTRUMENTS

Motivational Interviewing Treatment Integrity Codes (MITI; pronounced "mighty")

Description. The MITI is the gold standard for tracking adherence to MI. The MITI was designed for use in research, as well as clinical, settings. The measure allows supervisors, trainers, or trained researchers to rate helpers on two dimensions, behavior counts and global ratings. Behavior counts involve tallying everything the helper says and classifying them into codes indicating whether they are MI-adherent, filler, or non-MI-adherent statements. For example, coders tally the number of reflections, open questions, efforts at collaborative statements, confrontational statements (contraindicated), and provision of advising without permission (contraindicated). Global scores generated include Cultivating Change Talk, Softening Sustain Talk, Empathy, and Partnership. These four dimensions are rated on a 5-point scale when considering the session as a whole.

Potential Uses in Learning MI. A common training activity is submitting an audio recorded MI session for review by an experienced MI trainer. Learners can contract with MI trainers to evaluate their MI sessions and provide coaching sessions. Coaching is highly recommended in the MI community as a method of learning. Another training activity with the MITI involves listening to a tape that has already been coded by MI experts. This is a standard activity in the MI course that I teach to Master's in Social Work (MSW) students. I also have students code each other's work as they are learning MI. Although to my knowledge there is no scientific research confirming that coding leads to improved training outcomes, many MI trainers and practitioners vouch for the value of coding training in their learning processes.

Availability. At this writing, the most recent version of the MITI is publicly available from the University of New Mexico's Center on Substance Use, Alcohol, and Addiction (UNM CASAA) website. Coded and uncoded transcripts, as well as their accompanying audio recordings, are also available.

Working Alliance Inventory for Couples (WAI-CO)

Description. This is a self-report questionnaire that clients can complete. It is the couples' version of the widely used and researched Working Alliance Inventory (WAI). There are three sections to this instrument. First, there is a section where an individual can report on their alliance with a helper (21 items). Included in these items are ones that measure whether and to what extent the individual feels scapegoated by the family or views the family's problems systemically. Second, an individual can report on how they perceive their partner's alliance with the helper (21 items). Finally, the couple can report on their communal alliance with the helper (21 items).

Potential Uses in Learning MI. The WAI items appear to mostly map onto the concepts of engagement and partnership in the MITI. Other measures, such as the MITI or MISO, however, will be needed to evaluate helper efforts at eliciting change talk or sustain talk. The WAI-CO could be used in one's current practice with families to evaluate how well they are agreeing on goals. One unique feature of the measure is that it does also allow identification of whether the one or more members of the family believe in a systemic approach to solving their family's problems. Additionally, helpers can obtain multiple perspectives on how various family members view their and others' therapeutic alliances.

Availability. The WAI-CO is currently available online. You can obtain a copyright release by emailing *SPRexecutive@gmail.com* with the subject line "Limited Copyright Release for the WAI."

Motivational Interviewing with Significant Others (MISO)

Description. The MISO is a measure used to code audio-recorded MI sessions that include concerned significant others. It contains three global measures, including support, collaboration, and contemptuousness, as well as ten different behavior counts (e.g., significant other change talk).

Potential Uses for Learning MI. The MISO highlights current thinking about how to code change language from a concerned significant other (CSO) in relation to an identified client's target behavior. It could be used to code sessions where you are discussion the need for an identified client to make changes with a CSO. For example, you could use it to code a session of a helper talking with a parent about supporting their child losing weight if they are being seen in a wellness clinic.

Availability. At this writing, the most recent version of the MISO is publicly available by visiting the University of New Mexico's Center on Substance Use, Alcohol, and Addiction (UNM CASAA) website.

DEMONSTRATION VIDEOS AND AUDIO RECORDINGS

"My Father Also Hit Me" Videos

Description. These two brief videos are among my favorites for training students learning MI. One video shows impeccable MI, and an accompanying video shows the same client where the spirit of MMI is grossly violated. The case scenario involves a young man that was referred to parenting classes after an incident where he struck his child.

Potential Uses for Learning MI. In addition to the obvious family themes involved in this video, several teaching points can be demonstrated using it. First, by contrasting the two different counseling styles with an identical client, one can contrast the MI Spirit between the two tapes. Further, deconstruction can occur if you use the session transcripts and highlight the microskills used on the tape that are described in Chapter 2. Finally, I like this highlighting of the potential friction between female helpers and this male client based on his explicit statements about masculinity. These statements are a potential trap for confrontation, which is contraindicated in MI.

Availability. These videos are available for purchase from The Change Companies. See their website for additional details.

ASSESSMENT AND THERAPY MANUALS

GAIN Quick Manual

Description. This technical manual supports the use of the GAIN Q, a widely used and empirically validated assessment. The GAIN Quick takes approximately 30–45 minutes to administer. If the computer version of the instrument is used, users can automatically generate electronic or print copies of various reports, such as a formatted progress note and a personalized feedback report that can facilitate an MI session. There is a chapter included on using MI following the structured assessment, as discussed in Chapter 5 on engagement.

Potential Uses for Learning MI. Some learners find it helpful to have a structured feedback report when first learning MI. Although it is never wise to read long sections of a report to a client, it can be an aid to an otherwise conversational MI session.

Availability. The manual is available through Chestnut Health Systems, as is training on the GAIN Q instrument administration. Training on the CHOICE model, the MI session following the standardized assessment, is available by contacting me at *dougsmithconsulting@gmail.com*.

SOFT Training Manual

Description. A fully developed manual for the Strengths-Oriented Family Therapy program is available.

Potential Uses for Learning MI. It outlines both family-centered intake processes (SORT), as well as group sessions that can be used with parents and teens.

Availability. It is an unpublished document available by contacting the author (*dougsmithconsulting@gmail.com*).

Motivational Interviewing Assessment: Supervisory Tools for Enhancing Proficiency (MIA-STEP) Manual

Description. This treatment manual outlines how to do an "MI sandwich" where MI engages clients prior to and following a structured agency assessment.

Potential Uses for Learning MI. Several transcripts of sessions are available in both English and Spanish, which can be used for learning or training purposes. The manual may be beneficial to those tinkering with integrating MI into initial assessment processes.

Availability. The MIA-STEP manual is available free of charge. A publicly available copy is posted on the Motivational Interviewing Network of Trainers' (MINT) website.

Project MATCH Motivational Enhancement Therapy Manual

Description: This manual was used to deliver MI to individuals with alcohol use disorders.

Potential Uses for Learning MI. It outlines the MI model, as well as guidelines for significant other (SO) involvement. These SOs were typically family members.

Availability. It is available free of charge at on the United States National Institute of Alcoholism and Alcohol Abuse's website.

Project COMBINE Manual

Description. This manual was used to deliver combined behavior and pharmacological interventions to adults with alcohol use disorders.

Potential Uses for Learning MI. The manual outlines principles for significant other inclusion in treatment, including ways of vetting who may be the most supportive family member or significant other to include based on how supportive they are of goals of treatment.

Availability. The manual is free of charge and available on the United States National Institute of Alcoholism and Alcohol Abuse's website.

MINDFULNESS RESOURCES

The Center for Healthy Minds, University of Wisconsin–Madison

Description. This organization completes research on mindfulness, including studies on brain images and how mindfulness relates to compassion and empathy. They also developed a mobile app that can be used for practicing mindfulness.

Potential Uses for Learning MI. This resource can primarily be used for learning more about the research on how mindfulness may influence compassion and empathy. Also, their mobile application, Healthy Minds, may be used in attempts to increase one's focus before family sessions.

Availability. A number of press releases and descriptions of research studies exist on their website. Their website also has links and descriptions of their mobile app, Healthy Minds.

Jon Kabat-Zinn, Professor Emeritus at the University of Massachusetts

Description. Dr. Kabat-Zinn is one of the most well-recognized figures in the field of mindfulness meditation. He developed the Mindfulness-Based Stress Reduction (MSBR) program, has written numerous books on mindfulness, and has recorded a number of guided mindfulness meditation recordings.

Potential Uses for Learning MI. Compassion meditation may be a useful tool for preparing helpers to communicate the MI Spirit to clients.

Availability. A number of audio resources, YouTube videos of Dr. Kabat-Zinn, and books are available for learning compassion meditation.

LOCATING TRAINING

Motivational Interviewing Network of Trainers (MINT)

Description. MINT is an international organization of MI trainers dedicated to maintaining high training quality standards. Approximately 2,000 active members spread across the globe provide training and teaching, applying MI in a wide variety of settings. Among its members are many of the thought leaders on MI, including authors of books in The Guilford Press Applications of Motivational Interviewing series, to which this book belongs.

Membership in MINT is not an automatic guarantee of training quality. Although members initially must submit a recording demonstrating their expertise in MI as a practitioner and attend a MINT-sponsored Training of New Trainers (TNT) event, training skills take time to develop and hone.

MINT's Professional Development Committee, which I currently Co-Chair, is in the process of finalizing a trainer certification process. At present, about 75 of MINT's 2,000 members have been through this process and may use the title MINT Certified Trainer. To become a MINT Certified Trainer, one must be a MINT member in good standing for 2 or more years and submit a videotape of a training, which is then coded by MI trainers in MINT.

Potential Uses for Learning MI. One can review the list of current members by geographic area to select trainers, or to contact for coaching on MI. For those who have already received some training in MI and are interested in becoming MI trainers, they may find out more information about upcoming TNT events.

Availability. TNT events fill up quickly. To contact MINT about upcoming TNT events or available trainers, see their website.

References

Abar, C., & Turrisi, R. (2008). How important are parents during the college years? A longitudinal perspective of indirect influences parents yield on their college teens' alcohol use. *Addictive Behaviors, 33*(10), 1360–1368.

Abramson, L. Y., Metalsky, G. I., & Alloy, L. B. (1989). Hopelessness depression: A theory-based subtype of depression. *Psychological Review, 96*(2), 358–372.

Abughosh, S., Wang, X., Serna, O., Esse, T., Mann, A., Masilamani, S., . . . Fleming, M. (2017). A motivational interviewing intervention by pharmacy students to improve medication adherence. *Journal of Managed Care & Specialty Pharmacy, 23*(5), 549–560.

Adams, I., Braun, A., Hill, E., Al-Muhanna, K., Stigall, N., Lobb, J., . . . Spees, C. (2019). NP23 garden-based intervention for youth improves dietary and physical activity patterns, quality of life, family relationships, and indices of health. *Journal of Nutrition Education and Behavior, 51*(7, Suppl.), S20–S21.

Agliata, A. K., & Renk, K. (2008). College students' adjustment: The role of parent–college student expectation discrepancies and communication reciprocity. *Journal of Youth and Adolescence, 37*, 967–982.

American Association for Marriage and Family Therapy. (2004). Marriage and Family Therapy Core Competencies. Available at *www.coamfte.org/Documents/COAMFTE/Accreditation%20Resources/MFT%20Core%20Competencies%20(December%202004).pdf*.

American Association for Marriage and Family Therapy. (2015). *Code of Ethics*. Available at *www.aamft.org/Legal_Ethics/Code_of_Ethics.aspx*.

Amrhein, P. C., Miller, W. R., Yahne, C. E., Palmer, M., & Fulcher, L. (2003). Client commitment language during motivational interviewing predicts drug use outcomes. *Journal of Consulting and Clinical Psychology, 71*(5), 862.

Anderson, S. R., Tambling, R., Yorgason, J. B., & Rackham, E. (2019). The mediating role of the therapeutic alliance in understanding early discontinuance. *Psychotherapy Research, 29*(7), 882–893.

Anderson, V., Levin, H. S., & Jacobs, R. (2002). Executive functions after frontal lobe injury: A developmental perspective. In D. T. Stuss & R. T. Knight (Eds.), *Principles of frontal lobe function* (pp. 504–527). Oxford University Press.

Anton, R. F., O'Malley, S. S., Ciraulo, D. A., Cisler, R. A., Couper, D., Donovan, D. M., . . . COMBINE Study Research Group. (2006). Combined pharmacotherapies and behavioral interventions for alcohol dependence: The COMBINE study: A randomized controlled trial. *JAMA, 295*(17), 2003–2017.

Apodaca, T. R., Jackson, K. M., Borsari, B., Magill, M., Longabaugh, R., Mastroleo, N. R., & Barnett, N. P. (2016). Which individual therapist behaviors elicit client change talk and sustain talk in motivational interviewing? *Journal of Substance Abuse Treatment, 61*, 60–65.

Apodaca, T. R., Magill, M., Longabaugh, R., Jackson, K. M., & Monti, P. M. (2013). Effect of a significant other on client change talk in motivational interviewing. *Journal of Consulting and Clinical Psychology, 81*(1), 35–46.

Apodaca, T., Manuel, J. K., Moyers, T., & Amrhein, P. (2007). *Motivational Interviewing with Significant Others (MISO) coding manual.* Unpublished manuscript. Available at *https://casaa.unm.edu/assets/docs/miso.pdf*.

Aquilino, W. S. (2006). Family relationships and support systems in emerging adulthood. In J. J. Arnett & J. L. Tanner (Eds.), *Emerging adults in America: Coming of age in the 21st century.* (pp. 193–217). American Psychological Association.

Ariss, T., & Fairbairn, C. E. (2020). The effect of significant other involvement in treatment for substance use disorders: A meta-analysis. *Journal of Consulting and Clinical Psychology, 88*(6), 526–540.

Armstrong, S., Mendelsohn, A., Bennett, G., Taveras, E. M., Kimberg, A., & Kemper, A. R. (2018). Texting motivational interviewing: A randomized controlled trial of motivational interviewing text messages designed to augment childhood obesity treatment. *Childhood Obesity, 14*(1), 4–10.

Arnett, J. J. (2000). Emerging adulthood: A theory of development from the late teens through the twenties. *American Psychologist, 55*(5), 469–480.

Arnett, J. J. (2007). Emerging adulthood: What is it, and what is it good for? *Child Development Perspectives, 1*(2), 68–73.

Arnett, J. (2015). (Ed.). (2015). *The Oxford handbook of emerging adulthood.* Oxford University Press.

Arnett, J. J., Žukauskienė, R., & Sugimura, K. (2014). The new life stage of emerging adulthood at ages 18–29 years: Implications for mental health. *The Lancet Psychiatry, 1*(7), 569–576.

Audet, C. T., & Everall, R. D. (2010). Therapist self-disclosure and the therapeutic relationship: A phenomenological study from the client perspective. *British Journal of Guidance & Counselling, 38*(3), 327–342.

Baldwin, S. A., Christian, S., Berkeljon, A., & Shadish, W. R. (2012). The effects of family therapies for adolescent delinquency and substance abuse: A meta-analysis. *Journal of Marital and Family Therapy, 38*(1), 281–304.

Bamm, E. L., & Rosenbaum, P. (2008). Family-centered theory: origins, development, barriers, and supports to implementation in rehabilitation medicine. *Archives of Physical Medicine and Rehabilitation, 89*(8), 1618–1624.

Bandura, A. (1977). Self-efficacy: Toward a unifying theory of behavioral change. *Psychological Review, 84*(2), 191–215.

Barbato, A., & D'Avanzo, B. (2008). Efficacy of couple therapy as a treatment for depression: A meta-analysis. *Psychiatric Quarterly, 79*(2), 121–132.

Baucom, D. H., Sayers, S. L., & Sher, T. G. (1990). Supplementing behavioral marital therapy with cognitive restructuring and emotional expressiveness training: An outcome investigation. *Journal of Consulting and Clinical Psychology, 58*(5), 636–645.

Baumrind, D. (2005). Patterns of parental authority and adolescent autonomy. *New Directions for Child and Adolescent Development, 108*, 61–69.

Bean, M. K., Thornton, L. M., Jeffers, A. J., Gow, R. W., & Mazzeo, S. E. (2019). Impact of motivational interviewing on engagement in a parent-exclusive paediatric obesity intervention: Randomized controlled trial of NOURISH+MI. *Pediatric Obesity, 14*(4), e12484.

Beck, A. T., Rush, A. J., Shaw, B. F., & Emery, G. (1979). *Cognitive therapy of depression*. Guilford Press.

Beckman, M., Lindqvist, H., Öhman, L., Forsberg, L., Lundgren, T., & Ghaderi, A. (2022). Correspondence between practitioners' self-assessment and independent motivational interviewing treatment integrity ratings. *Frontiers in Psychology, 13*, 890579.

Belmontes, K. C. (2018). When family gets in the way of recovery: Motivational interviewing with families. *The Family Journal, 26*(1), 99–104.

Belsky, J., Jaffee, S., Hsieh, K.-H., & Silva, P. A. (2001). Child-rearing antecedents of intergenerational relations in young adulthood: A prospective study. *Developmental Psychology, 37*(6), 801.

Benish, S. G., Quintana, S., & Wampold, B. E. (2011). Culturally adapted psychotherapy and the legitimacy of myth: A direct-comparison meta-analysis. *Journal of Counseling Psychology, 58*(3), 279–289.

Berg, I. K. (1994). *Family-based services: A solution-focused approach*. Norton.

Berkel, C., Mauricio, A. M., Rudo-Stern, J., Dishion, T. J., & Smith, J. D. (2021). Motivational interviewing and caregiver engagement in the Family Check-Up 4 Health. *Prevention Science, 22*(6), 737–746.

Bibeau, M., Dionne, F., & Leblanc, J. (2016). Can compassion meditation contribute to the development of psychotherapists' empathy? A review. *Mindfulness, 7*(1), 255–263.

Blakely, K. M., Pytlik Zillig, L. M., & Speck, K. (2017). Applying motivational interviewing to parenting act mediation: The promise of the process. *The Nebraska Lawyer, January/February*, 31–36.

Blue, C. M., Arnett, M. C., Ephrem, H., Lunos, S., Ruoqiong, C., & Jones, R. (2020). Using motivational interviewing to reduce parental risk related behaviors for early childhood caries: A pilot study. *BMC Oral Health, 20*(1), 90.

Borrelli, B., Tooley, E. M., & Scott-Sheldon, L. A. J. (2015). Motivational interviewing for parent–child health interventions: A systematic review and meta-analysis. *Pediatric Dentistry, 37*(3), 254–265.

Bortolon, C. B., Moreira, T. C., Signor, L., Guahyba, B. L., Figueiro, L. R., Ferigolo, M., & Barros, H. M. (2017). Six-month outcomes of a randomized, motivational tele-intervention for change in the codependent behavior of family members of drug users. *Substance Use and Misuse, 52*(2), 164–174.

Bourke, E., Magill, M., & Apodaca, T. R. (2016). The in-session and long-term role of a significant other in motivational enhancement therapy for alcohol use disorders. *Journal of Substance Abuse Treatment, 64*, 35–43.

Briar-Lawson, K., Lawson, H. A., & Hennon, C. B. (2001). *Family-centered policies and practices: International implications.* Columbia University Press.

Bronfenbrenner, U. (1977). Toward an experimental ecology of human development. *American Psychologist, 32*(7), 513.

Cabral, R. R., & Smith, T. B. (2011). Racial/ethnic matching of clients and therapists in mental health services: A meta-analytic review of preferences, perceptions, and outcomes. *Journal of Counseling Psychology, 58*(4), 537–554.

Carr, A. (1990). Failure in family therapy: A catalogue of engagement mistakes. *Journal of Family Therapy, 12*(4), 371–386.

Carr, A. (2015). The evolution of systems theory. In T. L. Sexton & J. Lebow (Eds.), *Handbook of family therapy* (pp. 13–29). Routledge.

Carroll, K. M., Ball, S. A., Nich, C., Martino, S., Frankforter, T. L., Farentinos, C., . . . National Institute on Drug Abuse Clinical Trials Network. (2006). Motivational interviewing to improve treatment engagement and outcome in individuals seeking treatment for substance abuse: A multisite effectiveness study. *Drug and Alcohol Dependence, 81*(3), 301–312.

Caruthers, A. S., Van Ryzin, M. J., & Dishion, T. J. (2014). Preventing high-risk sexual behavior in early adulthood with family interventions in adolescence: Outcomes and developmental processes. *Prevention Science, 15*(1), 59–69.

Casey, B. J., & Jones, R. M. (2010). Neurobiology of the adolescent brain and behavior: Implications for substance use disorders. *Journal of the American Academy of Child & Adolescent Psychiatry, 49*(12), 1189–1201.

Chahal, N., Rush, J., Manlhiot, C., Boydell, K. M., Jelen, A., & McCrindle, B. W. (2017). Dyslipidemia management in overweight or obese adolescents: A mixed-methods clinical trial of motivational interviewing. *SAGE Open Medicine, 5*, 2050312117707152.

Child Welfare Information Gateway. (2017). *Infant safe haven laws.* U.S. Department of Health and Human Services, Children's Bureau. Available at www.childwelfare.gov/pubPDFs/safehaven.pdf#page=2&view= Who%20May%20Leave%20a%20Baby%20at%20Safe%20Haven.

Clawson, R. E., Davis, S. Y., Miller, R. B., & Webster, T. N. (2018). The case for insurance reimbursement of couple therapy. *Journal of Marital and Family Therapy, 44*(3), 512–526.

Colapinto, J. (1982). Structural family therapy. In A. M. Horne & M. M. Olsen (Eds.), *Family counseling and therapy.* F. E. Peacock.

Colapinto, J. (2016). Structural family therapy. In T. L. Sexton & J. Lebow (Eds.), *Handbook of family therapy: The science and practice of working with families and couples* (2nd ed., pp. 134–147). Routledge.

Commission on Accreditation for Marriage and Family Therapy Education. (2021). *Accreditation standards: Graduate & post-graduate marriage and family therapy training programs* (version 12.5). Retrieved from *www.coamfte.org*.

Connell, A., Dishion, T., Yasui, M., & Kavanagh, K. (2007). An adaptive approach to family intervention: Linking engagement in family-centered intervention to reductions in adolescent problem behavior. *Journal of Consulting and Clinical Psychology, 75*, 568–579.

Connell, A. M., McKillop, H. N., & Dishion, T. J. (2016). Long-term effects of the Family Check-Up in early adolescence on risk of suicide in early adulthood. *Suicide and Life-Threatening Behavior, 46*(S1), S15–S22.

Cordova, J. V., Fleming, C. J., Morrill, M. I., Hawrilenko, M., Sollenberger, J. W., Harp, A. G., . . . Wachs, K. (2014). The Marriage Checkup: A randomized controlled trial of annual relationship health checkups. *Journal of Consulting and Clinical Psychology, 82*(4), 592–604.

Cordova, J. V., Warren, L. Z., & Gee, C. B. (2001). Motivational interviewing as an intervention for at risk couples. *Journal of Marital and Family Therapy, 27*(3), 315–326.

Couture, S. J. (2006). Transcending a differend: Studying therapeutic processes conversationally. *Contemporary Family Therapy, 28*(3), 285–302.

Crocetti, E. (2017). Identity formation in adolescence: The dynamic of forming and consolidating identity commitments. *Child Development Perspectives, 11*(2), 145–150.

Cushing, C. C., Jensen, C. D., Miller, M. B., & Leffingwell, T. R. (2014). Meta-analysis of motivational interviewing for adolescent health behavior: Efficacy beyond substance use. *Journal of Consulting and Clinical Psychology, 82*, 1212–1218.

Czyz, E. K., King, C. A., & Biermann, B. J. (2019). Motivational interviewing-enhanced safety planning for adolescents at high suicide risk: A pilot randomized controlled trial. *Journal of Clinical Child & Adolescent Psychology, 48*(2), 250–262.

Dallacker, M., Hertwig, R., & Mata, J. (2019). Quality matters: A meta-analysis on components of healthy family meals. *Health Psychology, 38*(12), 1137.

D'Amico, E. J., Dickerson, D. L., Brown, R. A., Johnson, C. L., Klein, D. J., & Agniel, D. (2020). Motivational interviewing and culture for urban Native American youth (MICUNAY): A randomized controlled trial. *Journal of Substance Abuse Treatment, 111*, 86–99.

D'Amico, E. J., Houck, J. M., Hunter, S. B., Miles, J. N., Osilla, K. C., & Ewing, B. A. (2015). Group motivational interviewing for adolescents: Change talk and alcohol and marijuana outcomes. *Journal of Consulting and Clinical Psychology, 83*(1), 68–80.

D'Aniello, C., Piercy, F. P., Dolbin-MacNab, M. L., & Perkins, S. N. (2019). How clients of marriage and family therapists make decisions about therapy discontinuation and persistence. *Contemporary Family Therapy: An International Journal, 41*(1).

Dattilio, F. M. (2005). The critical component of cognitive restructuring in couples therapy: A case study. *Australian and New Zealand Journal of Family Therapy, 26*(2), 73–78.

Davis, E. E., Pitchford, N. J., & Limback, E. (2011). The interrelation between cognitive and motor development in typically developing children aged 4–11 years is underpinned by visual processing and fine manual control. *British Journal of Psychology, 102*(3), 569–584.

Davis, J. P., Smith, D. C., & Briley, D. A. (2017). Substance use prevention and treatment outcomes for emerging adults in non-college settings: A meta-analysis. *Psychology of Addictive Behaviors, 31*(3), 242–254.

Davoli, A. M., Broccoli, S., Bonvicini, L., Fabbri, A., Ferrari, E., D'Angelo, S., . . . Giorgi Rossi, P. (2013). Pediatrician-led motivational interviewing to treat overweight children: An RCT. *Pediatrics, 132*(5), e1236–e1246.

Dawson, A. M., Brown, D. A., Cox, A., Williams, S. M., Treacy, L., Haszard, J., . . . Taylor, R. W. (2014). Using motivational interviewing for weight feedback to parents of young children. *Journal of Pediatrics and Child Health, 50*(6), 461–470.

Del Re, A. C., Flückiger, C., Horvath, A. O., Symonds, D., & Wampold, B. E. (November 2012). Therapist effects in the therapeutic alliance–outcome relationship: A restricted-maximum likelihood meta-analysis. *Clinical Psychology Review, 32*(7), 642–649.

Denham, S., von Salisch, M., Olthof, T., Kochanoff, A., & Caverly, S. (2002). Emotional and social development in childhood. *Blackwell Handbook of Childhood Social Development*, 307–328.

Dennis, M. L., Titus, J. C., White, M. K., Unsicker, J. I., & Hodgkins, D. (2002). *Global Appraisal of Individual Needs—Initial (GAIN-I)*. Chestnut Health Systems.

de Shazer, S. (1988). *Clues. Investigating solutions in brief therapy.* Norton.

de Shazer, S., & Dolan, Y. (2012). *More than miracles: The state of the art of solution-focused brief therapy.* Routledge.

DeVargas, E. C., & Stormshak, E. A. (2020). Motivational interviewing skills as predictors of change in emerging adult risk behavior. *Professional Psychology: Research and Practice, 51*(1), 16–24.

de Vries, N. M., Staal, J. B., van der Wees, P. J., Adang, E. M., Akkermans, R., Olde Rikkert, M. G., & Nijhuis-van der Sanden, M. W. (2016). Patient-centred physical therapy is (cost?) effective in increasing physical activity and reducing frailty in older adults with mobility problems: A randomized controlled trial with 6 months follow-up. *Journal of Cachexia, Sarcopenia and Muscle, 7*(4), 422–435.

Diamond, G., & Liddle, H. A. (1996). Resolving a therapeutic impasse between parents and adolescents in multidimensional family therapy. *Journal of Consulting and Clinical Psychology, 64*(3), 481–488.

Diener, E. (1984). Subjective well-being. *Psychological Bulletin, 95*(3), 542–575.

Dishion, T. J., Brennan, L. M., Shaw, D. S., McEachern, A. D., Wilson, M. N., & Jo, B. (2014). Prevention of problem behavior through annual family check-ups in early childhood: Intervention effects from home to early elementary school. *Journal of Abnormal Child Psychology, 42*(3), 343–354.

Dishion, T. J., & Kavanagh, K. (2003). *Intervening in adolescent problem behavior: A family-centered approach.* Guilford Press.

Dishion, T. J., McCord, J., & Poulin, F. (1999). When interventions harm. Peer groups and problem behavior. *American Psychologist, 54*(9), 755–764.

Dishion, T. J., Nelson, S. E., & Kavanagh, K. (2003). The Family Check-Up with high-risk young adolescents: Preventing early-onset substance use by parent monitoring. *Behavior Therapy, 34*(4), 553–571.

Dishion, T. J., Shaw, D., Connell, A., Gardner, F., Weaver, C., & Wilson, M. (2008). The family check-up with high-risk indigent families: Preventing problem behavior by increasing parents' positive behavior support in early childhood. *Child Development, 79*(5), 1395–1414.

Dishion, T. J., & Stormshak, E. A. (2007). *Intervening in children's lives: An ecological, family-centered approach to mental health care.* American Psychological Association.

Döring, N., Ghaderi, A., Bohman, B., Heitmann, B. L., Larsson, C., Berglind, D., . . . Rasmussen, F. (2016). Motivational interviewing to prevent childhood obesity: A cluster RCT. *Pediatrics, 137*(5).

DuBose, K. D., & Dlugonski, D. (2018). Effect of a parental modeling intervention on parent and 1- to 5-year-old children's physical activity. *Translational Journal of the American College of Sports Medicine, 3*(21), 169.

Duncan, S., Goodyear-Smith, F., McPhee, J., Zinn, C., Grøntved, A., & Schofield, G. (2016). Family-centered brief intervention for reducing obesity and cardiovascular disease risk: A randomized controlled trial. *Obesity, 24*(11), 2311–2318.

Ellis, D. A., Idalski Carcone, A., Ondersma, S. J., Naar-King, S., Dekelbab, B., & Moltz, K. (2017). Brief computer-delivered intervention to increase parental monitoring in families of African American adolescents with type 1 diabetes: A randomized controlled trial. *Telemedicine and E-Health, 23*(6), 493–502.

Epstein, E. E., & McCrady, B. S. (1998). Behavioral couples treatment of alcohol and drug use disorders: Current status and innovations. *Clinical Psychology Review, 18*(6), 689–711.

Erickson, S. J., Gerstle, M., & Feldstein, S. W. (2005). Brief interventions and motivational interviewing with children, adolescents, and their parents in pediatric health care settings: A review. *Archives of Pediatrics & Adolescent Medicine, 159*(12), 1173–1180.

Erikson, E. H. (1993). *Childhood and society* (2nd ed.). Norton.

Faustino-Silva, D. D., Colvara, B. C., Meyer, E., Hugo, F. N., Celeste, R. K., & Hilgert, J. B. (2019). Motivational interviewing effects on caries prevention in children differ by income: A randomized cluster trial. *Community Dentistry and Oral Epidemiology, 47*(6), 477–484.

Felix, H. C., Narcisse, M. R., Long, C. R., English, E., Haggard-Duff, L., Purvis, R. S., & McElfish, P. A. (2019). The effect of family diabetes self-management education on self-care behaviors of Marshallese adults with type 2 diabetes. *American Journal of Health Behavior, 43*(3), 490–497.

Felix, H. C., Narcisse, M. R., Long, C. R., & McElfish, P. A. (2020). Effects of a family diabetes self-management education intervention on the patients' supporters. *Families, Systems, and Health, 38*(2), 121–129.

Fingerman, K. L., Cheng, Y. P., Wesselmann, E. D., Zarit, S., Furstenberg, F., & Birditt, K. S. (2012). Helicopter parents and landing pad kids: Intense parental support of grown children. *Journal of Marriage and Family, 74*(4), 880–896.

Fishbane, M. D. (2011). Facilitating relational empowerment in couple therapy. *Family Process, 50*(3), 337–352.

Flavell, J. H. (1999). Cognitive development: Children's knowledge about the mind. *Annual Review of Psychology, 50*(1), 21–45.

Fokas, K. F., Houck, J. M., & McCrady, B. S. (2020). Inside alcohol behavioral couple therapy (ABCT): In-session speech trajectories and drinking outcomes. *Journal of Substance Abuse Treatment, 118*, 108122.

Forgatch, M. S., & Patterson, G. R. (2010). Parent management training—Oregon model: An intervention for antisocial behavior in children and adolescents. In J. R. Weisz & A. E. Kazdin (Eds.), *Evidence-based psychotherapies for children and adolescents* (pp. 159–177). Guilford Press.

Fosco, G. M., Frank, J. L., Stormshak, E. A., & Dishion, T. J. (2013). Opening the "Black Box": Family Check-Up intervention effects on self-regulation that prevents growth in problem behavior and substance use. *Journal of School Psychology, 51*(4), 455–468.

Frey, A. J., Cloud, R. N., Lee, J., Small, J. W., Seeley, J. R., Feil, E. G., . . . Golly, A. (2011). The promise of motivational interviewing in school mental health. *School Mental Health, 3*, 1–12.

Fried, T. R. (2022). Giving up on the objective of providing goal-concordant care: Advance care planning for improving caregiver outcomes. *Journal of the American Geriatrics Society, 70*(10), 3006–3011.

Fried, T. R., Paiva, A. L., Redding, C. A., Iannone, L., O'Leary, J. R., Zenoni, M., . . . Rossi, J. S. (2021). Effect of the STAMP (Sharing and Talking About My Preferences) intervention on completing multiple advance care planning activities in ambulatory care: A cluster randomized controlled trial. *Annals of Internal Medicine, 174*(11), 1519–1527.

Friedlander, M. L., Escudero, V., Welmers-van de Poll, M. J., & Heatherington, L. (2018). Meta-analysis of the alliance–outcome relation in couple and family therapy. *Psychotherapy, 55*(4), 356–371.

Gaume, J., Gmel, G., Faouzi, M., & Daeppen, J. B. (2008). Counsellor behaviours and patient language during brief motivational interventions: A sequential analysis of speech. *Addiction, 103*(11), 1793–1800.

Ghaderi, A., Kadesjö, C., Björnsdotter, A., & Enebrink, P. (2018). Randomized effectiveness trial of the Family Check-Up versus internet-delivered parent training (iComet) for families of children with conduct problems. *Scientific Reports, 8*(1), Article 1.

Godley, S. H., Smith, J. E., Meyers, R. J., & Godley, M. D. (2016). *The adolescent community reinforcement approach: A clinical guide for treating substance use disorders*. Chestnut Health Systems.

Goodyear, M., Maybery, D., Reupert, A., Allchin, R., Fraser, C., Fernbacher, S., & Cuff, R. (2017). Thinking families: A study of the characteristics of the workforce that delivers family-focused practice. *International Journal of Mental Health Nursing, 26*(3), 238–248.

Gottman, J. S., & Gottman, J. M. (2015). *10 principles for doing effective couples therapy*. Norton.

Gray, T. D., Hawrilenko, M., & Cordova, J. V. (2020). Randomized controlled trial of the marriage checkup: Depression outcomes. *Journal of Marital and Family Therapy, 46*(3), 507–522.

Hamilton, S., Moore, A. M., Crane, D. R., & Payne, S. H. (2011). Psychotherapy dropouts: Differences by modality, license, and DSM-IV diagnosis. *Journal of Marital and Family Therapy, 37*(3), 333–343.

Harrison, R., Benton, T., Everson-Stewart, S., & Weinstein, P. (2007). Effect of motivational interviewing on rates of early childhood caries: A randomized trial. *Pediatric Dentistry, 29*(1), 16–22.

Hawkins, J. D., Catalano, R. F., & Miller, J. Y. (1992). Risk and protective factors for alcohol and other drug problems in adolescence and early adulthood: Implications for substance abuse prevention. *Psychological Bulletin, 112*(1), 64–105.

Heatherington, L., Friedlander, M. L., & Greenberg, L. (2005). Change process research in couple and family therapy: Methodological challenges and opportunities. *Journal of Family Psychology, 19*(1), 18–27.

Henggeler, S. W., & Schaeffer, C. M. (2019). Multisystemic Therapy®: Clinical procedures, outcomes, and implementation research. In B. H. Fiese, M. Celano, K. Deater-Deckard, E. N. Jouriles, & M. A. Whisman (Eds.), *APA handbook of contemporary family psychology: Family therapy and training* (pp. 205–220). American Psychological Association.

Herman-Giddens, M. E., Smith, J. B., Mittal, M., Carlson, M., & Butts, J. D. (2003). Newborns killed or left to die by a parent: A population-based study. *JAMA, 289*(11), 1425–1429.

Hettema, J., Steele, J., & Miller, W. R. (2005). Motivational interviewing. *Annual Review of Clinical Psychology, 1*, 91–111.

Hoeve, M., Dubas, J. S., Eichelsheim, V. I., Van der Laan, P. H., Smeenk, W., & Gerris, J. R. (2009). The relationship between parenting and delinquency: A meta-analysis. *Journal of Abnormal Child Psychology, 37*(6), 749–775.

Holtzman, M. (2008). Defining family: Young adults' perceptions of the parent–child bond. *Journal of Family Communication, 8*(3), 167–185.

Horvath, A. O., & Greenberg, L. S. (1989). Development and validation of the Working Alliance Inventory. *Journal of Counseling Psychology, 36*(2), 223–233.

Huitt, W., & Hummel, J. (2003). Piaget's theory of cognitive development. *Educational Psychology Interactive*, 3(2), 1–5.

Hunter-Reel, D., Witkiewitz, K., & Zweben, A. (2012). Does session attendance by a supportive significant other predict outcomes in individual treatment for alcohol use disorders? *Alcoholism: Clinical and Experimental Research*, 36(7), 1237–1243.

Janicke, D. M., Steele, R. G., Gayes, L. A., Lim, C. S., Clifford, L. M., Schneider, E. M., . . . Westen, S. (2014). Systematic review and meta-analysis of comprehensive behavioral family lifestyle interventions addressing pediatric obesity. *Journal of Pediatric Psychology*, 39(8), 809–825.

Johnston, L. D., O'Malley, P. M., Bachman, J. G., Schulenberg, J. E. & Miech, R. A. (2015). *Monitoring the Future national survey results on drug use, 1975–2014: Volume 2, College students and adults ages 19–55*. Institute for Social Research, The University of Michigan.

Kang, H. Y., & Gu, M. O. (2015). Development and effects of a motivational interviewing self-management program for elderly patients with diabetes mellitus. *Journal of Korean Academy of Nursing*, 45(4), 533–543.

Kao, T.-S. A., Ling, J., Vu, C., Hawn, R., & Christodoulos, H. (2023). Motivational interviewing in pediatric obesity: A meta-analysis of the effects on behavioral outcomes. *Annals of Behavioral Medicine*, kaad006.

Karakurt, G., Whiting, K., Van Esch, C., Bolen, S. D., & Calabrese, J. R. (2016). Couples therapy for intimate partner violence: A systematic review and meta-analysis. *Journal of Marital and Family Therapy*, 42(4), 567–583.

Karney, B. R., & Bradbury, T. N. (2000). Attributions in marriage: State or trait? A growth curve analysis. *Journal of Personality and Social Psychology*, 78(2), 295–309.

Kazantzis, N., Luong, H. K., Usatoff, A. S., Impala, T., Yew, R. Y., & Hofmann, S. G. (2018). The processes of cognitive behavioral therapy: A review of meta-analyses. *Cognitive Therapy and Research*, 42, 349–357.

Kelly, J. F., Greene, M. C., & Abry, A. (2021). A US national randomized study to guide how best to reduce stigma when describing drug-related impairment in practice and policy. *Addiction*, 116(7), 1757–1767.

Kelly, J. F., & Westerhoff, C. M. (2010). Does it matter how we refer to individuals with substance-related conditions? A randomized study of two commonly used terms. *International Journal of Drug Policy*, 21(3), 202–207.

Kiecolt-Glaser, J. K. (2018). Marriage, divorce, and the immune system. *American Psychologist*, 73(9), 1098.

Kierkegaard, S. (2014). *The concept of anxiety: A simple psychologically oriented deliberation in view of the dogmatic problem of hereditary sin*. Norton.

Knudson-Martin, C., McDowell, T., & Bermudez, J. M. (2019). From knowing to doing: Guidelines for socioculturally attuned family therapy. *Journal of Marital and Family Therapy*, 45(1), 47–60.

Kohlberg, L., & Hersh, R. H. (1977). Moral development: A review of the theory. *Theory into Practice*, 16(2), 53–59.

Kosovski, J., & Smith, D. C. (2011). Everybody hurts: Addiction drama and the family in the reality television show *Intervention*. *Substance Use and Misuse, 46,* 852–858.

Landry, S. H., Smith, K. E., & Swank, P. R. (2003). The importance of parenting during early childhood for school-age development. *Developmental Neuropsychology, 24*(2–3), 559–591.

Larsen, R. T., Korfitsen, C. B., Keller, C., Christensen, J., Andersen, H. B., Juhl, C., & Langberg, H. (2021). The MIPAM trial—Motivational Interviewing and Physical Activity Monitoring to enhance the daily level of physical activity among older adults—A randomized controlled trial. *European Review of Aging and Physical Activity, 18*(1), 12.

Laursen, B., & Collins, W. A. (2009). Parent–child relationships during adolescence. In R. M. Lerner & L. Steinberg (Eds.), *Handbook of adolescent psychology: Contextual influences on adolescent development* (3rd ed., pp. 3–42). Wiley.

Lee, C. S. (2025). *Motivational interviewing across cultures: Optimizing practice*. Guilford Press.

Lee, C. S., López, S. R., Hernández, L., Colby, S. M., Caetano, R., Borrelli, B., & Rohsenow, D. (2011). A cultural adaptation of motivational interviewing to address heavy drinking among Hispanics. *Cultural Diversity and Ethnic Minority Psychology, 17*(3), 317–324.

Lee, R. M., Draper, M., & Lee, S. (2001). Social connectedness, dysfunctional interpersonal behaviors, and psychological distress: Testing a mediator model. *Journal of Counseling Psychology, 48*(3), 310.

Lewis, T. F., & Osborn, C. J. (2004). Solution-focused counseling and motivational interviewing: A consideration of confluence. *Journal of Counseling & Development, 82*(1), 38–48.

Liddle, H. A., Dakof, G. A., Turner, R. M., Henderson, C. E., & Greenbaum, P. E. (2008). Treating adolescent drug abuse: A randomized trial comparing multidimensional family therapy and cognitive behavior therapy. *Addiction, 103*(10), 1660–1670.

Liddle, H. A., & Hogue, A. (2000). A family-based, developmental-ecological preventive intervention for high-risk adolescents. *Journal of Marital and Family Therapy, 26*(3), 265–279.

Lin, C. Y., Yaseri, M., Pakpour, A. H., Malm, D., Broström, A., Fridlund, B., . . . Webb, T. L. (2017). Can a multifaceted intervention including motivational interviewing improve medication adherence, quality of life, and mortality rates in older patients undergoing coronary artery bypass surgery? A multicenter, randomized controlled trial with 18-month follow-up. *Drugs & Aging, 34,* 143–156.

Lindenberger, U. (2001). Lifespan theories of cognitive development. In *International encyclopedia of the social and behavioral sciences* (pp. 8848–8854). Elsevier Science.

Lloyd, C. E., Duncan, C., & Cooper, M. (2019). Goal measures for psychotherapy: A systematic review of self-report, idiographic instruments. *Clinical Psychology: Science and Practice, 26*(3), Article e12281.

Longabaugh, R., & Wirtz, P. W. (Eds.). (2001). *Project MATCH hypotheses: Results and causal chain analyses* (No. 1). U.S. Department of Health and Human Services, Public Health Service, National Institutes of Health, National Institute on Alcohol Abuse and Alcoholism.

Luberto, C. M., Shinday, N., Song, R., Philpotts, L. L., Park, E. R., Fricchione, G. L., & Yeh, G. Y. (2018). A systematic review and meta-analysis of the effects of meditation on empathy, compassion, and prosocial behaviors. *Mindfulness, 9*(3), 708–724.

Lundahl, B. W., Kunz, C., Brownell, C., Tollefson, D., & Burke, B. L. (2010). A meta-analysis of motivational interviewing: Twenty-five years of empirical studies. *Research on Social Work Practice, 20*(2), 137–160.

Lyman, D. R., Braude, L., George, P., Dougherty, R. H., Daniels, A. S., Ghose, S. S., & Delphin-Rittmon, M. E. (2014). Consumer and family psychoeducation: Assessing the evidence. *Psychiatric Services, 65*(4), 416–428.

MacDonell, K., Brogan, K., Naar-King, S., Ellis, D., & Marshall, S. (2012). A pilot study of motivational interviewing targeting weight-related behaviors in overweight or obese African American adolescents. *Journal of Adolescent Health, 50*(2), 201–203.

MacNeil, A., Connolly, M. T., Salvo, E., Kimball, P. F., Rogers, G., Lewis, S., & Burnes, D. (2023). Use of motivational interviewing by advocates in the context of an elder abuse response intervention: The RISE project. *Journal of Family Violence*, 1–11.

Magill, M., Apodaca, T. R., Borsari, B., Gaume, J., Hoadley, A., Gordon, R. E., . . . Moyers, T. (2018). A meta-analysis of motivational interviewing process: Technical, relational, and conditional process models of change. *Journal of Consulting and Clinical Psychology, 86*(2), 140.

Manuel, J. K., Houck, J. M., & Moyers, T. B. (2012). The impact of significant others in motivational enhancement therapy: Findings from Project MATCH. *Behavioural and Cognitive Psychotherapy, 40*(3), 297–312.

Marcia, J. E. (1993). The ego identity status approach to ego identity. In J. E. Marcia, A. S. Waterman, D. R. Matteson, S. L. Archer, & J. L. Orlofsky (Eds.), *Ego identity: A handbook for psychosocial research* (pp. 3–21). Springer.

Martin, B. A., Chewning, B. A., Margolis, A. R., Wilson, D. A., & Renken, J. (2016). Med Wise: A theory-based program to improve older adults' communication with pharmacists about their medicines. *Research in Social and Administrative Pharmacy, 12*(4), 569–577.

Martino, S., Ball, S. A., Gallon, S. L., Hall, D., Garcia, M., Ceperich, S., . . . Hausotter, W. (2006) Motivational Interviewing Assessment: Supervisory Tools for Enhancing Proficiency. Salem, OR: Northwest Frontier Addiction Technology Transfer Center, Oregon Health and Science University. Available at *https://motivationalinterviewing.org/sites/default/files/mia-step.pdf*.

McAdams, C. R. III, Foster, V. A., Tuazon, V. E., Kooyman, B. A., Gonzalez, E., Grunhaus, C. M., . . . Wagner, N. J. (2018). In-session therapist actions for improving client retention in family therapy: Translating empirical research into clinical practice. *Journal of Family Psychotherapy, 29*(2), 142–160.

McCrady, B. S., Tonigan, J. S., Ladd, B. O., Hallgren, K. A., Pearson, M. R., Owens, M. D., & Epstein, E. E. (2019). Alcohol behavioral couple therapy: In-session behavior, active ingredients and mechanisms of behavior change. *Journal of Substance Abuse Treatment, 99*, 139–148.

McCrady, B. S., Wilson, A. D., Muñoz, R. E., Fink, B. C., Fokas, K., & Borders, A. (2016). Alcohol-focused behavioral couple therapy. *Family Process, 55*(3), 443–459.

McDowell, T., Knudson-Martin, C., & Bermudez, J. M. (2019). Third-order thinking in family therapy: Addressing social justice across family therapy practice. *Family Process, 58*(1), 9–22.

McElfish, P. A., Long, C. R., Kohler, P. O., Yeary, K. H., Bursac, Z., Narcisse, M. R., . . . Goulden, P. A. (2019). Comparative effectiveness and maintenance of diabetes self-management education interventions for Marshallese patients with type 2 diabetes: a randomized controlled trial. *Diabetes Care, 42*(5), 849–858.

McGoldrick, M., & Shibusawa, T. (2012). The family life cycle. In F. Walsh (Ed.), *Normal family processes: Growing diversity and complexity* (4th ed.). Guilford Press.

McPherson, K. E., Kerr, S., Casey, B., & Marshall, J. (2017). Barriers and facilitators to implementing functional family therapy in a community setting: Client and practitioner perspectives. *Journal of Marital and Family Therapy, 43*(4), 717–732.

Mehta, C. M., Arnett, J. J., Palmer, C. G., & Nelson, L. J. (2020). Established adulthood: A new conception of ages 30 to 45. *American Psychologist, 75*(4), 431–444.

Metcalfe, R. E., Matulis, J. M., Cheng, Y., & Stormshak, E. A. (2021). Therapeutic alliance as a predictor of behavioral outcomes in a relationally focused, family-centered telehealth intervention. *Journal of Marital and Family Therapy, 47*(2), 473484.

Miklavcic, J. J., Fraser, K. D., Ploeg, J., Markle-Reid, M., Fisher, K., Gafni, A., . . . Upshur, R. (2020). Effectiveness of a community program for older adults with type 2 diabetes and multimorbidity: A pragmatic randomized controlled trial. *BMC Geriatrics, 20*, 1–4.

Miller, W. R. (1983). Motivational interviewing with problem drinkers. *Behavioural and Cognitive Psychotherapy, 11*(2), 147–172.

Miller, W. R., Benefield, R. G., & Tonigan, J. S. (1993). Enhancing motivation for change in problem drinking: A controlled comparison of two therapist styles, *61*(3), 455–461.

Miller, W. R., Meyers, R. J., & Tonigan, J. S. (1999). Engaging the unmotivated in treatment for alcohol problems: A comparison of three strategies for intervention through family members. *Journal of Consulting and Clinical Psychology, 67*(5), 688–697.

Miller, W. R., & Rollnick, S. (2009). Ten things that motivational interviewing is not. *Behavioural and Cognitive Psychotherapy, 37*(2), 129–140.

Miller, W. R., & Rollnick, S. (2012). *Motivational interviewing: Helping people change* (3rd ed). Guilford Press.

Miller, W. R., & Rollnick, S. (2023). *Motivational interviewing: Helping people change and grow* (4th ed.). Guilford Press.

Miller, W. R., & Rose, G. S. (2015). Motivational interviewing and decisional balance: Contrasting responses to client ambivalence. *Behavioural and Cognitive Psychotherapy, 43*(2), 129–141.

Minuchin, S. (1974). *Families and family therapy*. Harvard University Press.

Moral, R. R., de Torres, L. A. P., Ortega, L. P., Larumbe, M. C., Villalobos, A. R., García, J. A. F., . . . Collaborative Group ATEM-AP Study. (2015). Effectiveness of motivational interviewing to improve therapeutic adherence in patients over 65 years old with chronic diseases: Aa cluster randomized clinical trial in primary care. *Patient Education and Counseling, 98*(8), 977–983.

Morris, M., Halford, W. K., & Petch, J. (2018). A randomized controlled trial comparing family mediation with and without motivational interviewing. *Journal of Family Psychology, 32*(2), 269–275.

Moyers, T. B., Rowell, L. N., Manuel, J. K., Ernst, D., & Houck, J. M. (2016). The motivational interviewing treatment integrity code (MITI 4): Rationale, preliminary reliability and validity. *Journal of Substance Abuse Treatment, 65*, 36–42.

Mukamuyango, J., Ingabire, R., Parker, R., Nyombayire, J., Easter, S. R., Wall, K. M., . . . Karita, E. (2020). Motivational interviewing to promote long acting reversible contraception among Rwandan couples wishing to prevent or delay pregnancy. *American Journal of Obstetrics and Gynecology, 222*(4S), S919.

Naar, S., & Safren, S. A. (2017). *Motivational interviewing and CBT: Combining strategies for maximum effectiveness*. Guilford Press.

Naar, S., & Suarez, M. (2021). *Motivational interviewing with adolescents and young adults* (2nd ed.). Guilford Press.

Nedjat-Haiem, F. R., Cadet, T. J., Amatya, A., Thompson, B., & Mishra, S. I. (2019). Efficacy of motivational interviewing to enhance advance directive completion in Latinos with chronic illness: A randomized controlled trial. *American Journal of Hospice and Palliative Medicine®, 36*(11), 980–992.

Nichols, M. P., & Davis, S. D. (2020). *The essentials of family therapy* (7th ed.). Pearson Education.

Nock, M. K., & Kazdin, A. E. (2005). Randomized controlled trial of a brief intervention for increasing participation in parent management training. *Journal of Consulting and Clinical Psychology, 73*(5), 872–879.

Norcross, J. C., Zimmerman, B. E., Greenberg, R. P., & Swift, J. K. (2017). Do all therapists do that when saying goodbye? A study of commonalities in termination behaviors. *Psychotherapy, 54*(1), 66–75.

O'Farrell, T. J., & Fals-Stewart, W. (2012). *Behavioral couples therapy for alcoholism and drug abuse*. Guilford Press.

O'Rourke, H. M., Collins, L., & Sidani, S. (2018). Interventions to address social connectedness and loneliness for older adults: A scoping review. *BMC Geriatrics, 18*(1), 1–13.

Pakpour, A. H., Gellert, P., Dombrowski, S. U., & Fridlund, B. (2015). Motivational interviewing with parents for obesity: An RCT. *Pediatrics, 135*(3), e644–e652.

Papp, P., Scheinkman, M., & Malpas, J. (2013). Breaking the mold: Sculpting impasses in couples' therapy. *Family Process, 52*(1), 33–45.

Park, M., Lee, M., Jeong, H., Jeong, M., & Go, Y. (2018). Patient-and family-centered care interventions for improving the quality of health care: A review of systematic reviews. *International Journal of Nursing Studies, 87*, 69–83.

Pedrelli, P., Nyer, M., Yeung, A., Zulauf, C., & Wilens, T. (2015). College students: Mental health problems and treatment considerations. *Academic Psychiatry, 39*, 503–511.

Perumalswami C., Burke J., Singer D., Malani P., Kirch M., Solway E., ... Skolarus L. (2021, April). *Older Adults' Experiences with Advance Care Planning. University of Michigan National Poll on Healthy Aging.* Available at http://hdl.handle.net/2027.42/167012.

Piaget, J. (1953). *The origin of intelligence in the child.* Routledge & Kegan Paul.

Piaget, J., & Inhelder, B. (1969). *The psychology of the child.* Basic Books.

Pinquart, M. (2014). Associations of general parenting and parent–child relationship with pediatric obesity: A meta-analysis. *Journal of Pediatric Psychology, 39*(4), 381–393.

Porter, S. A. (2010). *Safe Haven Infant Protection: Incidence of use and characteristics of surrendered infants and relinquishing users.* New Jersey Institute of Technology. Available at: https://digitalcommons.njit.edu/cgi/viewcontent.cgi?article=1249&context=dissertations.

Prins, S. J., Shefner, R. T., Kajeepeta, S., Levy, N., Esie, P., & Mauro, P. M. (2023). Longitudinal relationships among exclusionary school discipline, adolescent substance use, and adult arrest: Public health implications of the school-to-prison pipeline. *Drug and Alcohol Dependence, 251*, 110949.

Prochaska, J. O., & DiClemente, C. C. (1982). Transtheoretical therapy: Toward a more integrative model of change. *Psychotherapy: Theory, research & practice, 19*(3), 276–288.

Prochaska, J. O., DiClemente, C. C., & Norcross, J. C. (1992). In search of the structure of change. In Y. Klar, J. D. Fisher, J. M. Chinsky, & A. Nadler (Eds.), *Self change: Social psychological and clinical perspectives* (pp. 87–114). Springer.

Project MATCH Research Group. (1998). Matching alcoholism treatments to client heterogeneity: Project MATCH three-year drinking outcomes. *Alcoholism: Clinical and Experimental Research, 22*(6), 1300–1311.

Reid, W. J., & Crisafulli, A. (1990). Marital discord and child behavior problems: A meta-analysis. *Journal of Abnormal Child Psychology, 18*(1), 105–117.

Rice, F. P., & Dolgin, K. G. (2005). *The adolescent: Development, relationships and culture.* Pearson Education New Zealand.

Riedinger, V., Pinquart, M., & Teubert, D. (2017). Effects of systemic therapy on mental health of children and adolescents: A meta-analysis. *Journal of Clinical Child & Adolescent Psychology, 46*(6), 880–894.

Rogers, C. (1961). *On becoming a person: A therapist's view of psychotherapy.* Houghton Mifflin.

Rollnick, S., Kaplan, S. G., & Rutschman, R. (2016). *Motivational interviewing in schools: Conversations to improve behavior and learning.* Guilford Press.

Roseneil, S., & Budgeon, S. (2004). Cultures of intimacy and care beyond 'the family': Personal life and social change in the early 21st century. *Current Sociology, 52*(2), 135–159.

Rubak, S., Sandbæk, A., Lauritzen, T., & Christensen, B. (2005). Motivational interviewing: A systematic review and meta-analysis. *British Journal of General Practice, 55*(513), 305–312.

Saleebey, D. (2012). *The strengths perspective in social work practice* (6th ed.). Pearson.

Salyers, M. P., Garabrant, J. M., Luther, L., Henry, N., Fukui, S., Shimp, D., . . . Rollins, A. L. (2019). A comparative effectiveness trial to reduce burnout and improve quality of care. *Administration and Policy in Mental Health and Mental Health Services Research, 46*(2), 238–254.

Schertz, A., Herbeck Belnap, B., Chavanon, M. L., Edelmann, F., Wachter, R., & Herrmann-Lingen, C. (2019). Motivational interviewing can support physical activity in elderly patients with diastolic heart failure: Results from a pilot study. *ESC Heart Failure, 6*(4), 658–666.

Schofield, W. (2019). *Psychotherapy: The purchase of friendship.* Routledge.

Schulz, R., Beach, S. R., Czaja, S. J., Martire, L. M., & Monin, J. K. (2020). Family caregiving for older adults. *Annual Review of Psychology, 71,* 635–659.

Schwartz, R. P., Hamre, R., Dietz, W. H., Wasserman, R. C., Slora, E. J., Myers, E. F., . . . Resnicow, K. A. (2007). Office-based motivational interviewing to prevent childhood obesity: A feasibility study. *Archives of Pediatrics & Adolescent Medicine, 161*(5), 495–501.

Seedall, R. B., Holtrop, K., & Parra-Cardona, J. R. (2014). Diversity, social justice, and intersectionality trends in C/MFT: A content analysis of three family therapy journals, 2004–2011. *Journal of Marital and Family Therapy, 40*(2), 139–151.

Seligman, M. E. (1972). Learned helplessness. *Annual Review of Medicine, 23*(1), 407–412.

Serdarevic, M., & Lemke, S. (2013). Motivational interviewing with the older adult. International *Journal of Health Promotion, 15*(4), 240–249.

Shaw, D. S., Dishion, T. J., Supplee, L., Gardner, F., & Arnds, K. (2006). Randomized trial of a family-centered approach to the prevention of early conduct problems: 2-year effects of the family check-up in early childhood. *Journal of Consulting and Clinical Psychology, 74*(1), 1–9.

Sheidow, A. J., McCart, M. R., & Drazdowski, T. K. (2022). Family-based treatments for disruptive behavior problems in children and adolescents: An updated review of rigorous studies (2014–April 2020). *Journal of Marital and Family Therapy, 48*(1), 56–82.

Sibley, M. H., Graziano, P. A., Kuriyan, A. B., Coxe, S., Pelham, W. E., Rodriguez, L., . . . Ward, A. (2016). Parent–teen behavior therapy + motivational interviewing for adolescents with ADHD. *Journal of Consulting and Clinical Psychology, 84*, 699–712.

Slavet, J. D., Stein, L. A. R., Klein, J. L., Colby, S. M., Barnett, N. P., & Monti, P. M. (2005). Piloting the Family Check-Up with incarcerated adolescents and their parents. *Psychological Services, 2*(2), 123–132.

Smeerdijk, M., Keet, R., Dekker, N., van Raaij, B., Krikke, M., Koeter, M., . . . Linszen, D. (2012). Motivational interviewing and interaction skills training for parents to change cannabis use in young adults with recent-onset schizophrenia: A randomized controlled trial. *Psychological Medicine, 42*(8), 1627–1636.

Smeerdijk, M., Keet, R., Van Raaij, B., Koeter, M., Linszen, D., De Haan, L., & Schippers, G. (2015). Motivational interviewing and interaction skills training for parents of young adults with recent-onset schizophrenia and co-occurring cannabis use: 15-month follow-up. *Psychological Medicine, 45*(13), 2839–2848.

Smith, D. C. (Ed.). (2017). *Emerging adults and substance use disorder treatment: Developmental considerations and innovative approaches.* Oxford University Press.

Smith, D. C., Cleeland, L., & Dennis, M. L. (2010) Reasons for quitting among emerging adults and adolescents in substance use disorder treatment. *Journal of Studies on Alcohol and Drugs, 71*(3), 400–409.

Smith, D. C., Davis, J. P., Ureche, D. J., & Dumas, T. M. (2016). Six month outcomes of a peer-enhanced community reinforcement approach for emerging adults with substance misuse: A preliminary study. *Journal of Substance Abuse Treatment, 61*, 66–73.

Smith, D. C., & Hall, J. A. (2007). Strengths oriented referral for teenagers (SORT): Giving balanced feedback to teens and families. *Health and Social Work, 32*(1), 69–72.

Smith, D. C., & Hall, J. A. (2008). Parenting style and adolescent clinical severity: Findings from two substance abuse treatment studies. *Journal of Social Work Practice in the Addictions, 8*(4), 440–463.

Smith, D. C., & Hall, J. A. (2010). Implementing evidence-based multiple-family groups with adolescent substance abusers. *Social Work with Groups, 33*, 1–17.

Smith, D. C., Hall, J. A., Jang, M., & Arndt, S. (2009). Therapist adherence to a motivational-interviewing intervention improves treatment entry for substance-misusing adolescents with low problem perception. *Journal of Studies on Alcohol and Drugs, 70*(1), 101–105.

Smith, D. C., Hall, J. A., Williams, J. K., An, H., Gotman, N. (2006) Comparative efficacy of family and group treatment for adolescent substance abuse. *The American Journal on Addictions, 15*(6), 131–136.

Smith, J. E., & Meyers, R. J. (2007). *Motivating substance abusers to enter treatment: Working with family members.* Guilford Press.

Sotero, L., & Relvas, A. P. (2021). Dropout versus retention in family therapy: How are they associated with behavioral manifestations of the therapeutic alliance? *Contemporary Family Therapy, 43,* 320–328.

Spirito, A., Sindelar-Manning, H., Colby, S. M., Barnett, N. P., Lewander, W., Rohsenow, D. J., & Monti, P. M. (2011). Individual and family motivational interventions for alcohol-positive adolescents treated in an emergency department: Results of a randomized clinical trial. *Archives of Pediatrics & Adolescent Medicine, 165*(3), 269–274.

Sprenkle, D. H. (2012). Intervention research in couple and family therapy: A methodological and substantive review and an introduction to the special issue. *Journal of Marital and Family Therapy, 38*(1), 3–29.

Sprenkle, D. H., Davis, S. D., & Lebow, J. L. (2009). *Common factors in couple and family therapy: The overlooked foundation for effective practice.* Guilford Press.

Starks, T. J. (2022). *Motivational interviewing with couples: A framework for behavior change developed with sexual minority men.* Oxford University Press.

Starks, T. J., Adebayo, T., Kyre, K. D., Millar, B. M., Stratton, M. J., Gandhi, M., & Ingersoll, K. S. (2022a). Pilot randomized controlled trial of motivational interviewing with sexual minority male couples to reduce drug use and sexual risk: The couples health project. *AIDS and Behavior,* 1–18.

Starks, T. J., Doyle, K. M., Stewart, J. L., Bosco, S. C., & Ingersoll, K. S. (2022b). Development of Motivational Interviewing Treatment Integrity (MITI) fidelity codes assessing motivational interviewing with couples. *AIDS and Behavior, 26*(1), 13–20.

Starks, T. J., Millar, B. M., Doyle, K. M., Bertone, P., Ohadi, J., & Parsons, J. T. (2018). Motivational interviewing with couples: A theoretical framework for clinical practice illustrated in substance use and HIV prevention intervention with gay male couples. *Psychology of Sexual Orientation and Gender Diversity, 5*(4), 490–502.

Steinberg, L. (2001). We know some things: Parent–adolescent relationships in retrospect and prospect. *Journal of Research on Adolescence, 11*(1), 1–19.

Steinberg, L. (2008). A social neuroscience perspective on adolescent risk-taking. *Developmental Review, 28,* 78–106.

Stone, A. L., Becker, L. G., Huber, A. M., & Catalano, R. F. (2012). Review of risk and protective factors of substance use and problem use in emerging adulthood. *Addictive Behaviors, 37*(7), 747–775.

Stormshak, E., Caruthers, A., Chronister, K., DeGarmo, D., Stapleton, J., Falkenstein, C., . . . Nash, W. (2019). Reducing risk behavior with family-centered prevention during the young adult years. *Prevention Science, 20*(3), 321–330.

Stormshak, E. A., Connell, A., & Dishion, T. J. (2009). An adaptive approach to family-centered intervention in schools: Linking intervention engagement to academic outcomes in middle and high school. *Prevention Science, 10*(3), 221–235.

Stormshak, E. A., Connell, A. M., Véronneau, M.-H., Myers, M. W., Dishion, T. J., Kavanagh, K., & Caruthers, A. S. (2011). An ecological approach to promoting early adolescent mental health and social adaptation: Family-centered intervention in public middle schools. *Child Development, 82*(1), 209–225.

Stormshak, E. A., DeGarmo, D., Garbacz, S. A., McIntyre, L. L., & Caruthers, A. (2021). Using motivational interviewing to improve parenting skills and prevent problem behavior during the transition to kindergarten. *Prevention Science, 22*(6), 747–757.

Strom, R. E., & Boster, F. J. (2007). Dropping out of high school: A meta-analysis assessing the effect of messages in the home and in school. *Communication Education, 56*(4), 433–452.

Szapocznik, J., & Williams, R. A. (2000). Brief strategic family therapy: Twenty-five years of interplay among theory, research and practice in adolescent behavior problems and drug abuse. *Clinical Child and Family Psychology Review, 3*(2), 117–134.

Tambling, R. B. (2012). A literature review of therapeutic expectancy effects. *Contemporary Family Therapy, 34*(3), 402–415.

Tambling, R. B., & Johnson, L. N. (2008). The relationship between stages of change and outcome in couple therapy. *The American Journal of Family Therapy, 36*(3), 229–241.

Tambling, R. B., & Ketring, S. A. (2014). The R-URICA: A confirmatory factor analysis and a revision to the URICA. *Contemporary Family Therapy, 36*(1), 108–119.

Tambling, R. R., Hynes, K. C., & D'Aniello, C. (2020). Are barriers to psychotherapy treatment seeking indicators of social determinants of health? A critical review of the literature. *The American Journal of Family Therapy*, 1–16.

Tambling, R. R., & Johnson, L. N. (2019). Predictive validity of the R-URICA. *Psychology and Psychotherapy: Theory, Research and Practice, 92*(3), 407–421.

Tellez, M., Myers Virtue, S., Neckritz, S., Bhoopathi, V., Hernández, M., & Shearer, B. (2019). Motivational interviewing and oral health education: Experiences from a sample of elderly individuals in North and Northeast Philadelphia. *Special Care in Dentistry, 39*(2), 201–207.

Toth, S. L., & Cicchetti, D. (1999). Developmental psychopathology and child psychotherapy. In S. W. Russ & T. H. Ollendick (Eds.), *Handbook of psychotherapies with children and families* (pp. 15–44). Springer.

Trillingsgaard, T., Fentz, H. N., Hawrilenko, M., & Cordova, J. V. (2016). A randomized controlled trial of the Marriage Checkup adapted for private practice. *Journal of Consulting and Clinical Psychology, 84*(12), 1145.

Tryon, G. S., Birch, S. E., & Verkuilen, J. (2018). Meta-analyses of the relation of goal consensus and collaboration to psychotherapy outcome. *Psychotherapy, 55*(4), 372–383.

Tse, M. M., Vong, S. K., & Tang, S. K. (2013). Motivational interviewing and exercise programme for community-dwelling older persons with chronic pain: A randomised controlled study. *Journal of Clinical Nursing, 22*(13–14), 1843–1856.

Tucker, S. J., Ytterberg, K. L., Lenoch, L. M., Schmit, T. L., Mucha, D. I., Wooten, J. A., . . . Mongeon Wahlen, K. J. (2013). Reducing pediatric overweight: Nurse-delivered motivational interviewing in primary care. *Journal of Pediatric Nursing, 28*(6), 536–547.

Turrisi, R., Larimer, M. E., Mallett, K. A., Kilmer, J. R., Ray, A. E., Mastroleo, N. R., . . . Montoya, H. (2009). A randomized clinical trial evaluating a combined alcohol intervention for high-risk college students. *Journal of Studies on Alcohol and Drugs, 70*(4), 555–567.

Turrisi, R., Wiersma, K. A., & Hughes, K. K. (2000). Binge-drinking-related consequences in college students: Role of drinking beliefs and mother–teen communications. *Psychology of Addictive Behaviors, 14*(4), 342.

Tuvemo Johnson, S., Anens, E., Johansson, A. C., & Hellström, K. (2021). The Otago Exercise Program with or without motivational interviewing for community-dwelling older adults: A 12-month follow-up of a randomized, controlled trial. *Journal of Applied Gerontology, 40*(3), 289–299.

Venner, K. L., Feldstein, S. W., & Tafoya, N. (2006). *Native American motivational interviewing: Weaving Native American and western practices.* [Unpublished Manuscript]. University of New Mexico.

Vonnegut, K. (1985). How to write with style. In B. S. Fuess Jr. (Ed.), *How to use the power of the printed word.* Doubleday.

Wagner, C. C., & Ingersoll, K. S. (2012). *Motivational interviewing in groups.* Guilford Press.

Waite, L. J. (1995). Does marriage matter? *Demography, 32*(4), 483–507.

Walls, T. A., Fairlie, A. M., & Wood, M. D. (2009). Parents do matter: A longitudinal two-part mixed model of early college alcohol participation and intensity. *Journal of Studies on Alcohol and Drugs, 70*(6), 908–918.

Walsh, F. (2012). The new normal: Diversity and complexity in 21st-century families. In F. Walsh (Ed.), *Normal family processes: Growing diversity and complexity* (4th ed., pp. 3–27). Guilford Press.

Wampold, B. E., & Imel, Z. E. (2015). *The great psychotherapy debate: The evidence for what makes psychotherapy work.* Routledge.

Wang, Y., Jiao, Y., Nie, J., O'Neil, A., Huang, W., Zhang, L., . . . Woodward, M. (2020). Sex differences in the association between marital status and the risk of cardiovascular, cancer, and all-cause mortality: A systematic review and meta-analysis of 7,881,040 individuals. *Global Health Research and Policy, 5*(1), 1–16.

Waraan, L., Siqveland, J., Hanssen-Bauer, K., Czjakowski, N. O., Axelsdóttir, B., Mehlum, L., & Aalberg, M. (2023). Family therapy for adolescents with depression and suicidal ideation: A systematic review and meta-analysis. *Clinical Child Psychology and Psychiatry, 28*(2), 831–849.

Weinstein, P., Harrison, R., & Benton, T. (2004). Motivating parents to prevent caries in their young children: One-year findings. *The Journal of the American Dental Association, 135*(6), 731–738.

White, H. R., McMorris, B. J., Catalano, R. F., Fleming, C. B., Haggerty, K. P., & Abbott, R. D. (2006). Increases in alcohol and marijuana use during the transition out of high school into emerging adulthood: The effects of leaving home, going to college, and high school protective factors. *Journal of Studies on Alcohol, 67*(6), 810–822.

Whiteman, S. D., McHale, S. M., & Crouter, A. C. (2011). Family relationships from adolescence to early adulthood: Changes in the family system following firstborns' leaving home. *Journal of Research on Adolescence, 21*(2), 461–474.

Windsor, L. C, Smith, D. C., Bennett, K., M. and Gibbons, F. X. (2018). Substance use disorder treatments: Addressing the needs of emerging adults from privileged and marginalized backgrounds. In D. C. Smith (Ed.), *Emerging adults and substance use disorder treatment: Developmental considerations and innovative approaches* (pp. 96–118). Oxford University Press.

Wood, M. D., Fairlie, A. M., Fernandez, A. C., Borsari, B., Capone, C., Laforge, R., & Carmona-Barros, R. (2010). Brief motivational and parent interventions for college students: A randomized factorial study. *Journal of Consulting and Clinical Psychology, 78*(3), 349–361.

Wood, M. D., Read, J. P., Mitchell, R. E., & Brand, N. H. (2004). Do parents still matter? Parent and peer influences on alcohol involvement among recent high school graduates. *Psychology of Addictive Behaviors, 18*(1), 19.

Wood, N. D., Crane, D. R., Schaalje, G. B., & Law, D. D. (2005). What works for whom: A meta-analytic review of marital and couples therapy in reference to marital distress. *The American Journal of Family Therapy, 33*(4), 273–287.

Woodin, E. M., Sotskova, A., & O'Leary, K. D. (2012). Do motivational interviewing behaviors predict reductions in partner aggression for men and women? *Behaviour Research and Therapy, 50*(1), 79–84.

World Health Organization. (2024). Adolescent health. Available at *www.who.int/health-topics/adolescent-health#tab=tab_1*.

Wysocki, T., Harris, M. A., Buckloh, L. M., Mertlich, D., Lochrie, A. S., Taylor, A., ... White, N. H. (2008). Randomized, controlled trial of behavioral family systems therapy for diabetes: Maintenance and generalization of effects on parent–adolescent communication. *Behavior Therapy, 39*(1), 33–46.

Zimmerman, M. A. (2000). Empowerment theory. In J. Rappaport & E. Seidman (Eds.), *Handbook of community psychology* (pp. 43–63). Kluwer Academic.

Index

Note. *f*, *t*, or *n* following a page number indicates a figure, table, or note.

Ability statements
   evoking change talk and, 63–65, 64*t*
   overview, 57–59, 58*t*
   redundant change talk and, 70
   spotlighting change talk and, 67*t*
Acceptance. *See also* MI Spirit
   attending to the MI Spirit and, 25–27, 26*t*
   evoking change talk and, 62
   overlap among MI Spirit dimensions and, 38
   overview, 17, 23, 26*t*, 33–34, 38
Action planning, 70–71
Action stage of change, 8
Activation statements
   evoking change talk and, 63–65, 64*t*
   family-level equipoise and, 104, 107
   overview, 58*t*, 60
   redundant change talk and, 70
   spotlighting change talk and, 67*t*
Addiction, 8, 16. *See also* Substance use
Adolescents. *See also* Children; Developmental stages; Parenting; Young adults
   family-centered care and, 5, 6, 12–13
   MI with families with, 173–180, 176*t*–178*t*
   primacy of the family and, 4
Adults. *See* Established adults; Older adults; Young adults

Affirmations. *See also* OARS skills; ROARS skills
   cultural considerations and, 41
   engagement and, 128, 130, 132, 138
   family-level change talk and, 116
   family-level equipoise and, 103, 104, 106–107
   family-level ROARS and, 93, 99
   focusing task and, 145
   overview, 18, 49–50
   planning task and, 150
   scaling questions and, 59
   termination and, 157
Alcohol-focused behavioral couples therapy (ABCT), 195
Ambivalence. *See also* Sustain talk
   defining a target behavior and, 55, 56
   detecting, 56–66, 58*t*, 64*t*
   engagement and, 124, 125–134, 125*f*
   equipoise and, 19
   established and older adults and, 188–189
   evocation and, 62–63, 148
   expertise and, 31
   family systems perspectives and, 77–78
   family-level ROARS and, 93–95
   four tasks of MI and, 22
   history of MI and, 16
   integration of MI with family-centered care and, 84, 86, 90

231

Ambivalence *(cont.)*
  lack of change as, 55–56
  normalizing, 16, 56
  overview, 11, 23, 54–55, 71
  reasons for, 124
  reflections and, 45, 46
  resolving, 16–17, 126–127, 129–134
  ROARS skills and, 42
  solution-focused family therapy and, 86
  spotlighting change talk and, 66, 68
Amplified reflection, 64*t*, 128, 134. *See also* Reflections
Assessment, 122–124, 125*f*, 138–140
Autonomy
  adolescents and, 174–175
  coerced families and, 151
  engagement and, 123–124, 127, 128, 133
  established and older adults and, 188
  evoking task and, 148
  family-level equipoise and, 106–107
  motivational sendoffs and, 155
  open questions and, 48
  overlap among MI Spirit dimensions and, 38
  planning task and, 150, 151
  respecting, 23
  termination and, 158–160, 163
  young adults and, 183, 186–187

Behavior, 6, 7, 71, 84–86, 172, 179–180, 182–183. *See also* Target behavior
Behavioral couples therapy, 86
Behavioral multifamily group work, 88
Bias, 28, 35, 155
Boundaries, 30, 82–83, 136
Brief motivational intervention (BMI), 186
Brief refocusing summaries, 51, 52*t*. *See also* Reflective summaries
Brief strategic family therapy, 88

Case management services, 6, 88–89, 90
Center for Health Minds, University of Wisconsin–Madison, 207
Change, 6–7, 11, 31, 55–56. *See also* Change talk
Change talk. *See also* Family-level change talk; OARS skills; Sustain talk
  categories of, 57–60, 58*t*
  engagement and, 124, 138, 140
  evoking task and, 62–66, 64*t*, 146–147, 148
  in family work, 108–120, 113*f*, 117*f*
  family-level equipoise and, 102–108, 105*f*, 107*f*
  family-level ROARS and, 93–95
  focusing task and, 145
  interdependence of change language and, 118
  issues when listening for, 60–62
  overview, 18–19, 23, 57, 71, 100–101
  redundant change talk, 70
  simultaneous change and sustain language, 61–62
  solution-focused family therapy and, 87–88
  spotlighting, 66–71, 67*t*
  strategies for eliciting, 63–65, 64*t*
  transitioning to action planning and, 70–71
Change talk summaries, 51, 52*t*. *See also* Change talk; Reflective summaries; Summaries
Checking questions, 49. *See also* Questions
Child protection services, 12, 137–138
Children, 167, 168–173, 170*t*–171*t*. *See also* Adolescents; Developmental stages; Parenting
Clarity, 40–41, 42
Client-centered approaches, 27–28. *See also* Family-centered care
Clinicians. *See* Helpers
Closed questions, 49. *See also* Questions
Coerced families, 151, 161–162
Cognition, 84–86, 197
Cognitive restructuring, 86
Cognitive-behavioral family therapy, 82, 84–86
Cognitive-behavioral therapy (CBT), 16, 84–86, 194–195
Collaborative open question, 78. *See also* Open questions; Questions
Collaborative process. *See also* Partnership
  attending to the MI Spirit and, 27
  collaborative goal selection and, 143
  evoking task and, 148
  expert trap and, 30–31
  focusing task and, 144, 145
  overview, 11, 32–33
  planning task and, 151
College-age adults. *See* Young adults
Commitment statements
  evoking change talk and, 63–65, 64*t*
  overview, 58*t*, 60
  redundant change talk and, 70
  spotlighting change talk and, 67*t*

Index

Commitment to change, 155–157, 158, 161t
Communication, 4, 10, 14, 29–30
Community reinforcement approach, 86
Community reinforcement approach with family training (CRAFT) model, 126, 156–157
Compassion. *See also* MI Spirit
   attending to the MI Spirit and, 25–27, 26t
   ecological family therapies and, 90
   evoking task and, 148
   family engagement and, 138
   overlap among MI Spirit dimensions and, 38
   overview, 17, 23, 26t, 34–36, 38, 101
   reflections and, 43
   threats to, 35–36
Complex reflections. *See also* Reflections
   engagement and, 127, 128, 130, 131–132, 134
   evoking task and, 146
   family systems perspectives and, 78
   family-level change talk and, 114, 116
   family-level equipoise and, 103, 106
   family-level ROARS and, 94
   focusing task and, 145
   overview, 45–46
   planning task and, 150
Confidence ruler, 64t. *See also* Scaling questions
Conflict, family. *See* Relationships
Contemplation stage of change, 8
Core elements of MI, 17–19. *See also* Change talk; MI Spirit; Microcounseling skills
Coronary care, 191, 192t, 194, 201
Couple distress. *See* Marital distress; Relationships
Couples therapy, 109
Criminal justice context, 137–138
Cultural factors, 41, 42, 136–137, 182

DARN CAT mnemonic. *See also* Ability statements; Activation statements; Change talk; Commitment statements; Desire statements; Need statements; Reasons statements; Sustain talk; Taking steps statements
   evoking change talk and, 63–65, 64t
   issues when listening for change and sustain talk, 60–62

   overview, 57–60, 58t
   spotlighting change talk and, 66, 67t
Decisional balance exercise, 69
Desire statements
   evoking change talk and, 63–65, 64t
   overview, 57, 58t
   redundant change talk and, 70
   spotlighting change talk and, 67t
Developmental stages. *See also* Children; Older adults; Parenting
   adolescents, 173–180, 176t–178t
   compassion and, 35
   established adults, 188–196, 192t–193t
   family life cycles and, 79–80
   older adults, 188–190, 196–199
   overview, 167
   ROARS skills and, 41, 42
   school-age children, 172–173
   young adults, 181–187, 185t
   young children, 168–173, 170t–171t
Diabetes, 7, 191, 192t–193t, 194, 201
Double-sided reflections. *See also* Reflections
   engagement and, 128, 130
   evoking change talk and, 63, 65–66
   family-level ROARS and, 94–95, 96t
   planned uneasy terminations, 158
   planning task and, 149, 150
Dropping out of treatment. *See* Leaving care abruptly

Early childhood, 168. *See also* Children
Ecological family therapies, 82, 88–90
Elder care. *See* Older adults
Emerging adults. *See* Young adults
Empathy
   change and sustain talk and, 18–19
   ecological family therapies and, 90
   engagement and, 131–133, 134, 135, 137, 141
   evocation and, 62, 63, 146
   family systems perspectives and, 78
   family-level change talk and, 114
   family-level ROARS and, 98
   focusing task and, 145
   MI with families with young adults, 184
   planning task and, 149, 150, 151
   reflections and, 43
   ROARS skills and, 42
   tasks of MI and, 142–144
   termination and, 155, 160–162, 161t

Index

Empowerment. *See also* MI Spirit; Power
  attending to the MI Spirit and, 25–27, 26t
  overlap among MI Spirit dimensions and, 38
  overview, 11, 17, 23, 26t, 36–37, 38
Ending of services. *See* Leaving care abruptly; Motivational sendoffs; Termination
End-of-session summaries, 51, 52t, 160–162. *See also* Reflective summaries; Summaries
Engagement. *See also* Engaging task; Treatment retention
  assessment and, 122–124
  challenges in family-centered care and, 7–9
  engaging families, 134–136
  evaluating, 138–140
  family engagement and social justice and, 136–138
  family-centered care and, 14
  focusing task and, 145
  overview, 121, 140–141, 142–144
  partnership and, 32
  reluctant family members, 129–134
  resolving ambivalence and, 11
  tasks in engaging families, 121–129, 125f
  therapeutic alliances and, 9
  treatment retention and, 7–10, 11, 14
Engaging task, 22–23, 142–144, 153. *See also* Engagement
Equipoise. *See also* Family-level equipoise
  in family work, 100–108, 105f, 107f, 120
  family-level ROARS and, 96t
  overview, 19
  spotlighting change talk and, 69
Established adults, 188–190, 192t–193t, 199–200, 201. *See also* Parenting
Ethical issues, 69, 126–127
Evocation, 145, 147, 184, 188. *See also* Evoking task
Evocative complex reflections, 78, 130, 134. *See also* Complex reflections; Evocation; Reflections
Evoking task. *See also* Evocation
  engaging reluctant family members, 132
  exercise related to, 152
  family systems perspectives and, 77–78
  family-level change talk and, 115, 116
  family-level equipoise and, 103, 106
  family-level ROARS and, 93–94
  overview, 22–23, 71, 142–144, 146–149, 153
  partnership and, 32
  pivoting and, 92
  planning task and, 149
  redundant change talk and, 70
  solution-focused family therapy and, 87–88
  spotlighting change talk and, 66–71, 67t
  transitioning from sustain talk toward evoking change talk and, 62–66, 64t
Exception finding questions, 87. *See also* Questions
Expectations, 55–56
Expertise, 27–31, 32, 148

Family check-up (FCU)
  adolescents and, 175, 176t–178t, 179–180
  sequencing engagement and assessment and, 123–124
  Young Adult Family Check-Up (YA-FCU), 184, 185t
  young adults and, 184, 185t
Family conflict. *See* Relationships
Family engagement, 134–141. *See also* Engagement
Family life cycle, 79–80. *See also* Developmental stages
Family management treatment, 179
Family mediation, 102–108, 105f, 107f
Family motivational intervention (FMI), 181
Family psychoeducation, 6, 7
Family roles, 182
Family sculpting, 158
Family systems perspectives, 28–29, 75–79, 82. *See also* Family-centered care
Family therapy, 4–5, 6, 82–90. *See also* Family-centered care
Family-centered care. *See also* Integration of MI with family-centered care
  adolescents and, 173–180, 176t–178t
  challenges in, 4, 7–11
  concepts in, 75–82
  delivery of, 24–25
  ecological family therapies, 88–90
  engagement and, 125–129, 125f
  established adults and, 188–190, 192t–193t, 199–200

expertise and, 27–31
family life cycles and, 79–80
family models and, 6–7
family systems perspectives and, 76–79
homeostasis and, 81–82
models of family work and, 82–90
older adults and, 188–190, 196–200, 201
opportunities for using MI in, 12–13
overview, 4–6, 11, 14, 75, 90, 100, 167, 187
resources for, 203–208
school-age children and, 172–173
systems perspective and, 28–29
young adults and, 181–187, 185*t*
young children and, 168–173, 170*t*–171*t*
Family-level affirmations, 93, 99. *See also* Affirmations; Family-level ROARS
Family-level change talk, 100–101, 108–120, 113*f*, 117*f*. *See also* Change talk
Family-level equipoise, 101–108, 105*f*, 107*f*, 109, 120, 134. *See also* Equipoise
Family-level open questions, 95, 97, 147, 150. *See also* Family-level ROARS; Open questions
Family-level reflections. *See also* Family-level ROARS; Reflections
complex reflections, 145
double-sided reflections, 95, 96*t*
evoking task and, 146, 147
overview, 93–95, 96*t*, 99
reflective summaries, 97
simple reflection, 115
Family-level ROARS. *See also* ROARS skills
exercise related to, 99, 119, 152
interdependence of change language and, 118
overview, 91, 92, 93–97, 96*t*, 98, 100
Family-level target behavior (FTB). *See also* Target behavior
change talk and, 112–116, 113*f*
defining, 111
exercise related to, 119
interdependence of change language and, 118
overview, 117, 117*f*
Feedback loops, 76, 78, 163
Fixing reflex, 29, 132–133
Focusing task, 22–23, 68, 142–146, 152, 153

GAIN Q instrument, 205–206
Global Appraisal of Individual Needs, 123–124
Goals, 70–71, 86, 148, 183. *See also* Planning task

Helpers. *See also* Therapeutic relationship
acceptance and, 33–34
benefits of learning MI, 9–11
change and sustain talk and, 18–19
compassion and, 35–36
engagement and, 121–129, 125*f*, 135–136, 138–140, 141
evoking task and, 148
expert trap and, 27–31
family life cycles and, 79–80
family systems perspectives and, 76–77
family-centered care and, 6
four tasks of MI and, 22
language and, 55–56
motivational sendoffs and, 155
overview, 24–25
parenting styles and, 30–31
partnership and, 32–33
ROARS skills and, 39–42
unplanned terminations and, 163
History of MI, 15–16
Homeostasis, 81–82, 83
Humanistic approaches, 28, 55, 82

Identified client
change talk and, 109–110
engagement and, 125*f*, 126
family systems perspectives and, 76
family-level equipoise and, 108
MI with established and older adults and, 200, 201
overview, 5–6
Impasse, 158
Importance ruler, 64*t*. *See also* Scaling questions
Infancy, 168, 169. *See also* Children
Insight-oriented therapies, 86
Integration of MI with family-centered care. *See also* Family-centered care
cognitive-behavioral family therapy and, 86
ecological family therapies and, 90
family life cycles and, 79–80
family systems perspectives and, 75–79
MI with older adults and, 197–199
opportunities for, 12–13

Index

Integration of MI with family-centered care (cont.)
  overview, 4–6, 11, 90
  resources for, 203–208
  solution-focused family therapy and, 87–88
  structural family therapy and, 84
Interdependence, 116, 118

Kabat-Zinn, Jon, 207–208
Key question, 70. See also Questions

Language
  ambivalence and, 55–56
  evoking change talk and, 62, 63, 71
  myth acceptance and, 29–30
  ROARS skills and, 40
  solution-focused family therapy and, 87
  spotlighting change talk and, 66
Learned helplessness, 37
Learning theory, 84–86
Leaving care abruptly. See also Termination; Treatment retention
  challenges in family-centered care and, 7–9
  engagement and, 121, 138
  exercise related to, 164
  expertise and, 31
  family-centered care and, 14
  language and, 154n
  motivational sendoffs and, 154–155, 160–163
  overview, 164
  planned successful terminations, 155–157
Lifespan approach to families, 79–80. See also Developmental stages
Listening
  attending to the MI Spirit and, 27
  engagement and, 121, 122–123, 137
  integration of MI with family-centered care and, 84
  issues when listening for change and sustain talk, 60–62
  overview, 142
  pivoting and, 92
  reflective listening, 23, 43–46, 46t
Loving-kindness meditations, 35

Maintenance stage of change, 9
Mandated treatment plans, 151, 161–162
Marginalized families, 37, 136–138
Marital distress, 6, 7, 12, 83. See also Relationships
Marriage Checkup (MC), 190–191
Mechanisms of change. See Change
Mediation, family, 102–108, 105f, 107f
Medications, 196, 197
Meditations, 35, 207–208
Mental health, 6, 7, 35, 179, 181
MI Spirit. See also Acceptance; Compassion; Empowerment; Partnership
  attending to, 25–27, 26t
  family-level equipoise and, 104
  open questions and, 48
  overlap among dimensions of, 38
  overview, 17, 20–22, 23, 24–25, 38
  ROARS skills and, 42
Micro-counseling skills. See also OARS skills
  equipoise and, 101
  evoking change talk and, 63–65, 64t
  overview, 18, 23, 91, 98
  ROARS skills and, 42
Middle childhood. See Adolescents; Children
Midlife. See Established adults
Mindfulness, 35, 207–208
Mindfulness-Based Stress Reduction (MSBR) program, 207–208
Miracle question, 87. See also Questions
Motivation
  evoking change talk and, 65–66
  family systems perspectives and, 77
  family-level ROARS and, 93–95, 98
  integration of MI with family-centered care and, 87–88
  overview, 154
  spotlighting change talk and, 66
Motivational enhancement therapy (MET), 86, 109–110, 194–195
Motivational Interviewing Assessment: Supervisory Tools for Enhancing Proficiency (MIA-STEP) protocol, 123–124, 206
Motivational interviewing (MI) in general
  benefits of learning MI, 9–11
  four tasks of, 22–23
  history of MI, 15–16
  opportunities for using in family-centered care, 12–13
  overview, 11, 16–22, 23

Motivational Interviewing Network of
    Trainers (MINT), 5, 208
Motivational Interviewing Skills Code
    (MISC) instrument, 200
Motivational Interviewing Treatment
    Integrity (MITI) codes, 186, 200,
    203–204
Motivational Interviewing with Significant
    Others (MISO) measure, 108,
    204–205
Motivational sendoffs. *See also* Termination
    exercise related to, 164
    overview, 154–155, 164
    planned successful terminations,
        155–157
    planned uneasy terminations, 158–160,
        161*t*
    unplanned terminations, 160–163
Multidimensional family therapy, 88
Multifamily groups, 180
Multilevel change talk, 112–113, 113*f*. *See
    also* Change talk
Multilevel target behavior (MTB). *See also*
    Target behavior
    exercise related to, 119
    family-level change talk and, 114–116
    interdependence of change language and,
        118
    overview, 111, 117, 117*f*
Multipurpose statements, 42, 149
Multisystemic family therapy, 88
"My Father Also Hit Me" video, 205
Myth acceptance, 29–30

Need statements
    evoking change talk and, 63–65, 64*t*
    overview, 58*t*, 59
    redundant change talk and, 70
    spotlighting change talk and, 67*t*

OARS skills, 18–19, 20–22, 39. *See also*
    Affirmations; Change talk; Family-
    level ROARS; Open questions;
    Reflections; ROARS skills; Summaries
Obesity, 4, 6, 172, 179
Older adults. *See also* Developmental stages
    family-centered care and, 6, 13
    overview, 188–190, 196–199, 201
    practice and research recommendations,
        199–200
    primacy of the family and, 4

Open questions. *See also* OARS skills;
    Questions; ROARS skills
    engagement and, 127–128, 131, 132
    evoking change talk and, 64*t*, 65–66,
        146, 147
    family systems perspectives and, 78
    family-level change talk and, 113, 115,
        116
    family-level equipoise and, 103, 104,
        106–107
    family-level ROARS and, 94, 95, 97
    focusing task and, 145
    overview, 18, 47–49
    planning task and, 149, 150, 151
    redundant change talk and, 70
    scaling questions and, 59
    termination and, 155, 157

Parent training model, 86
Parent-based intervention (PBI), 186
Parent–child relationships. *See*
    Relationships
Parenting. *See also* Adolescents; Children;
    Developmental stages
    acceptance and, 33–34
    adolescents, 173–180, 176*t*–178*t*
    expert trap and, 30–31
    overview, 4, 167
    school-age children, 172–173
    structural family therapy and, 83
    styles of, 30–31
    young children, 168–173, 170*t*–171*t*
Parsimony, 40–41
Partnership. *See also* MI Spirit; Therapeutic
    relationship
    attending to the MI Spirit and, 25–27,
        26*t*
    empowerment and, 37
    engagement and, 127–128
    engaging reluctant family members, 132
    family-level change talk and, 113
    open questions and, 48
    overlap among MI Spirit dimensions
        and, 38
    overview, 17, 23, 26*t*, 32–33, 38
    planning task and, 150, 151
    ROARS skills and, 42
Pediatric obesity. *See* Obesity
Personal change talk, 111–113, 113*f*. *See
    also* Change talk
Personal responsibility views, 35–36

Personal target behaviors, 111, 117f, 118. *See also* Target behavior
Pivoting
   evoking task and, 146
   family-level change talk and, 110–111
   family-level equipoise and, 102, 104–107, 105f, 107f
   family-level ROARS and, 93–95, 98
   overview, 91–92
Planning task
   evoking task and, 147
   exercise related to, 152
   overview, 22–23, 142–144, 149–151, 153
   transitioning to action planning and, 70–71
Power, 32. *See also* Empowerment
Precontemplation stage of change, 8, 143
Premature focus trap, 144, 146
Preparation stage of change, 8
Preschool ages, 168, 169, 172. *See also* Children
Presenting problems. *See* Target behavior
Process theories, 143
Professionals. *See* Helpers
Project COMBINE manual, 207
Project MATCH, 86, 109–110, 194–195, 206–207
Psychiatric services. *See* Mental health
Psychodynamic models, 82, 86
Psychoeducation, family, 6, 7
Punishment, 84–85

Question–answer trap, 47–48
Questions. *See also* Open questions
   compared to reflections, 45, 46t
   family systems perspectives and, 78
   family-level equipoise and, 106–107
   family-level ROARS and, 94, 98
   key question, 70
   question–answer trap and, 47–48
   scaling questions, 58–59, 64t, 65
   sequencing engagement and assessment and, 122–123
   solution-focused family therapy and, 87

Reasons statements
   evoking change talk and, 63–65, 64t
   family-level equipoise and, 103
   overview, 58t, 59
   redundant change talk and, 70
   spotlighting change talk and, 67t

Redundant change talk, 70. *See also* Change talk
Reflections. *See also* Complex reflections; OARS skills
   culturally accurate reflections, 137
   engagement and, 127, 130, 131–132, 134
   evocation and, 63, 64t, 65–66, 146, 147
   family life cycles and, 79–80
   family systems perspectives and, 78
   family-level change talk and, 114, 115
   family-level equipoise and, 104, 106–107
   family-level ROARS and, 93–95, 96t, 98, 99
   integration of MI with family-centered care and, 84
   language and, 40–41
   overview, 18, 43–46, 46t
   pivoting and, 92
   planning task and, 149, 151
   questions and, 49
   redundant change talk and, 70
   reflective listening, 23, 43–46, 46t
   reflective summaries, 51, 52t, 97
   scaling questions and, 59
   termination and, 155, 157, 158
   transitioning to action planning and, 70–71
Reflective listening, 23, 43–46, 46t. *See also* Listening; Reflections; ROARS skills
Reflective summaries, 51, 52t, 97. *See also* Reflections; ROARS skills; Summaries
Reinforcement
   cognitive-behavioral family therapy and, 84–85
   engaging reluctant family members, 133
   evoking task and, 146, 147, 148
   family-level change talk and, 114–115, 116
   family-level equipoise and, 102–108, 105f, 107f
   focusing task and, 145
   overview, 66–71, 67t, 77–78
   planning task and, 149, 150
Relationships. *See also* Marital distress
   established adults and, 190–191, 192t–193t, 201
   family conflict and, 12–13
   family-centered care and, 7
   marital/couple distress, 6, 7, 12, 83
   parent–child relationships, 183–184
   young adults and, 186

Reluctance, 11, 127–134, 161–162. *See also* Ambivalence
Resistance, 32, 48, 55–56, 77–78
Responsibility, 35–36
Risky behaviors, 179–180, 182, 183. *See also* Substance use
ROARS skills. *See also* Affirmations; Change talk; Family-level ROARS; OARS skills; Open questions; Reflections; Summaries
  evoking change talk and, 64*t*, 65
  MI with established and older adults and, 200
  open questions, 47–49
  overview, 39, 51, 53, 91, 98
  pivoting and, 91–92
  reflections, 43–46, 46*t*, 51
  spotlighting change talk and, 66
  strategic use of, 42
  use of, 40–42
Rogers, Carl, 27–28

Safety, 9, 148
Scaling questions, 58–59, 64*t*, 65, 70, 87. *See also* Questions
Scapegoating, 83
School-age children, 172–173. *See also* Children
Sculpting techniques, 158
Secondary personal target behavior, 111, 117, 117*f*, 118. *See also* Target behavior
Sendoffs, motivational. *See* Motivational sendoffs
Senior citizens. *See* Older adults
Seven Challenges model, 180
Sexual wellness, 190–191, 192*t*–193*t*, 201
Simple reflections. *See* Reflections
SMART goals, 86
Social factors, 182
Social justice, 136–138
Solution-focused family therapy, 82, 86–88
Spirit of MI. *See* MI Spirit
Spotlighting change talk, 66–71, 67*t*, 77–78. *See also* Change talk; Reinforcement
Stage theories, 143
Stages-of-change model, 8–9, 143
Stigma, 35, 37
Strengths, 87, 88, 179
Strengths-Oriented Family Therapy (SOFT), 88, 178*t*, 180, 206
Strengths-Oriented Referral for Teen (SORT), 123–124
Structural family therapy, 38, 82–84
Substance use
  addiction, 8, 16
  adolescents and, 179–180
  ecological family therapies and, 89
  established adults and, 194–196, 201
  family-centered care and, 6
  history of MI and, 15–16
  integrating MI with family-centered care and, 5
  language and, 55
  older adults and, 201
  primacy of the family and, 4
  stigma and, 11*n*
  young adults and, 181, 183, 184, 186
Summaries, 18, 51, 52*t*, 97. *See also* OARS skills; Reflective summaries; ROARS skills
Superfluous engagement trap, 144
Supervision, 61*n*, 143
Sustain talk. *See also* Ambivalence; Change talk
  categories of, 57–60, 58*t*
  engagement and, 124, 130, 131
  family-level change talk and, 109, 114, 115
  family-level ROARS and, 93–95
  issues when listening for, 60–62
  overview, 18–19, 57, 71
  questions and, 49
  simultaneous change and sustain language, 61–62
  solution-focused family therapy and, 87–88
  transitioning from toward evoking change talk, 62–66, 64*t*
Systemic family therapy, 82. *See also* Family systems perspectives

Taking steps statements
  evoking change talk and, 63–65, 64*t*
  family-level equipoise and, 107
  overview, 58*t*, 60
  redundant change talk and, 70
  spotlighting change talk and, 67*t*
  transitioning to action planning and, 70–71

Index

Target behavior. *See also* Family-level target behavior (FTB); Planning task
  engaging reluctant family members, 132–133
  evocation and, 71, 148
  family-level change talk and, 110–111, 116–117, 117f
  interdependence of change language and, 118
  overview, 7, 19, 55, 56
  spotlighting change talk and, 66
Tasks of MI, 22–23, 141–144, 152, 153. *See also* Engaging task; Evoking task; Focusing task; Planning task
Tentative language, 63, 66, 134. *See also* Language
Termination. *See also* Motivational sendoffs
  challenges in family-centered care and, 7–9
  engagement and, 121, 138
  exercise related to, 164
  expertise and, 31
  family-centered care and, 14
  overview, 164
  planned successful terminations, 155–157
  planned uneasy terminations, 158–160, 161t
  unplanned terminations, 160–163
Therapeutic relationship. *See also* Helpers; Partnership
  benefits of learning MI, 9–10
  challenges in family-centered care and, 9
  empowerment and, 37
  engagement and, 121
  evaluating engagement and, 138, 140
  evocation and, 71, 148
  family-centered care and, 14
  overview, 33, 91–92
Therapists. *See* Helpers
Toddlerhood, 168, 169. *See also* Children
Training programs, 24–25, 34–35, 208
Transition points, 79–80, 81. *See also* Developmental stages; Family life cycle
Transtheoretical model of behavioral change, 8–9, 143
Treatment planning, 122, 151. *See also* Planning task
Treatment retention, 7–10, 11, 14. *See also* Engagement; Leaving care abruptly
Triangulation, 133–134
Twelve-step facilitation therapy (TSF), 16, 194–195

Values, 33–34, 183, 199–200
Voice tone, 42

Working Alliance Inventory for Couples (WAI-CO), 204

Young Adult Family Check-Up (YA-FCU), 184, 185t
Young adults, 4, 173, 181–187, 185t
Young children. *See* Children